ADRENAL FATIGUE DIET

Reset your Energy, balance your Hormones, and Boost your Serotonin, Dopamine, and Oxytocin

(Including more than 50 recipes to boost your energy, neurotransmitters, and hormone levels)

By

Margaret A. Davis

Version 1.1

Published by HMPL Publishing at KDP

Get to know your publisher and his work at:

http://happyhealthygreen.life

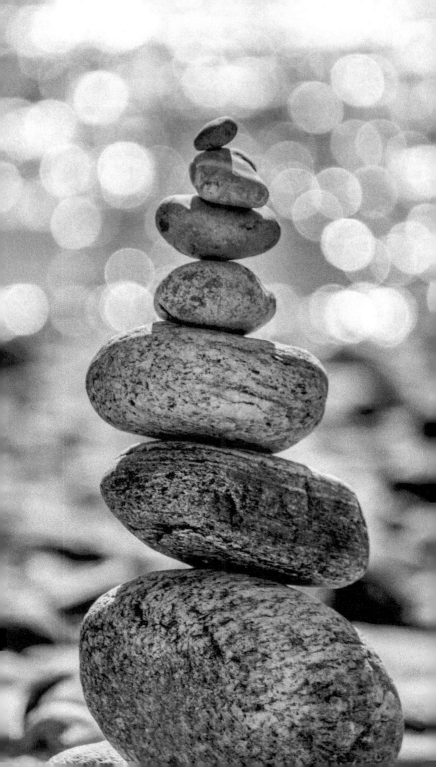

INTRODUCTION

Adrenal fatigue. Adrenal exhaustion. Adrenal burnout. Adrenal apathy. These interchangeable terms have become quite popular lately, and for good reason. Millions of people throughout the world deal with this condition.

The human brain is a highly complex, developed mass of soft nervous tissue. Even though it weighs only 3 pounds, this is where your feelings, drives, and motivations find their origin. Our brains are protected by the so-called cranium. The cranium is responsible for providing a protective shell to shield your delicate grey matter from outside forces.

Our skull and cranium do not guarantee full protection for the brain; things that could affect the condition of our grey mass from inside the body are excluded. This is both the responsibility and the psychological condition of the individual. Have you ever heard of the quotation "you are what you eat"? Nutrition, exercise, and sleep all have a major effect on our brain's condition and its everyday functions.

In this book, we will address common issues that deplete our energy levels and focus, and influence our everyday performance in a negative way. We will cover well-known issues like adrenal fatigue, neurotransmitter imbalances, brain fog, and other conditions that prevent you from firing all cylinders at full force.

Ultimately, you are responsible for what you put in your body and what you put your mind to. The way you treat your body and brain enables you to create and think clearly, and is of major importance to other essential cognitive functions.

In this book, you will learn how you can nurse your brain more effectively and regain your energy and mood. A change in your diet and daily habits, and the implementation of a healthier lifestyle, will help you break free from the chains of dizziness and unhappiness.

ADRENAL FATIGUE

How do you feel every morning when you wake up, get back from work, or are about to start something that really means something to you? Do you feel energized, refreshed, and highly motivated? Are you able to think with a clear head? Or have your days felt like a burden with frequent mood swings and depression? Although the problems might find their roots in different causes, your body and brain is not functioning the way they should.

To avoid potential setbacks in daily life and achieve your long-term goals, you want your body and brain to function the best they can. It is important to know that the most quintessential factor in improving your health and neurological performance goals involves eating a healthy diet that supplies you with the essential nutrients that your body needs to perform. Whole foods, healthy fats, and proteins are just mere examples; we will delve deeper into nutrition and its effect on your body.

In addition, the chemicals produced in your brain, better known as neurotransmitters, produce energy, help focus, and cause emotions. Since not everybody suffers from adrenal fatigue, brain fog, or direct effects of an insufficient diet, the book also covers various tips for balancing and increasing neurotransmitter levels in the brain.

Simply put, the adrenal fatigue diet comes down to eating the right foods to regulate both physical and mental functions and neurotransmitter levels in your brain, as well as help you improve the way you think, feel, and behave. It is recommended that you opt for organic ingredients as often as possible as these products contain less pesticides, artificial conditions, etc.

Your Goal is to reboot your energy levels and set yourself up for a sustainable lifestyle that includes a healthy brain with excellent mental functioning.

It should be known that the human brain uses far more energy than any other part of the body. By consuming the right foods full of quality nutrients, you will 'reset' your energy. In addition, you will balance your neurotransmitter levels that improves the overall functioning and performance of both your body and brain.

This book will give you some insight into how your brain works, how it runs at full speed, and how it is the central station of both your energy and individual happiness. When you finish reading this book, you will have a much better understanding regarding your brain and personal source of energy. Understanding is the first step towards change; this will then reflect as a better life with increased performance through this energy reset diet.

Obviously, understanding means very little without proper implementation. We have included many detailed, nutrient-rich and delicious recipes in this book. In the print version, you will even find a diet plan to guide your personal performance to the highest level.

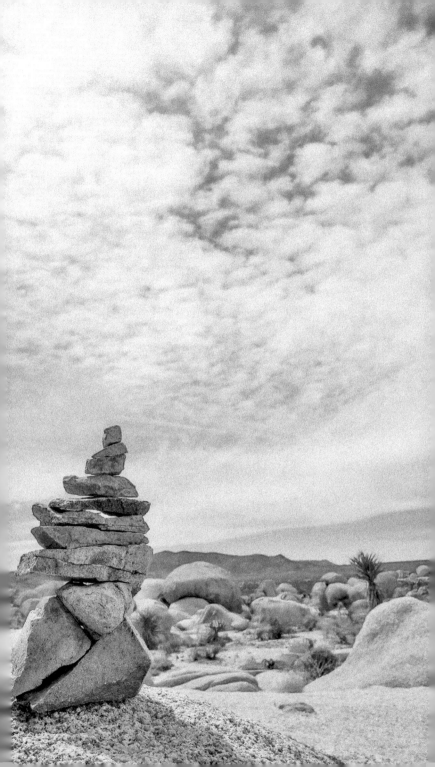

CONTENTS

DISCLAIMER

The recipes provided in this report are for informational purposes only and are not intended to provide dietary advice. A medical practitioner should be consulted before making any changes in diet. Additionally, recipe cooking times may require adjustment depending on age and quality of appliances. Readers are strongly urged to take all precautions to ensure ingredients are fully cooked and safe to consume in order to avoid the dangers of food borne viruses. The recipes and suggestions provided in this book are solely the opinion(s) of the author(s). The author and publisher do not take any responsibility for any consequences that may result due to following the instructions provided in this book.

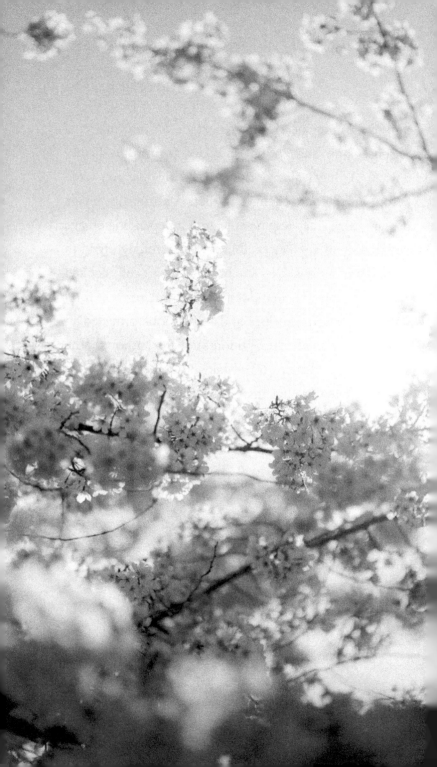

What Is Adrenal Fatigue

First, let us go over what the adrenals are. Your adrenals (or adrenal glands/stress glands) are two small glands that sit right on top of each kidney. You may not even know that they exist, but believe it or not, they are constantly working in the background when you are feeling exhausted. They typically weigh less than a grape at approximately 4 grams each and are just about the size of a walnut. Despite their size, they are incredibly powerful; some would say they are the foundation of health. Although small, their function in the human body is of utmost importance- that is, management of stress.

The adrenal glands have two parts: the outer adrenal cortex and the inner adrenal medulla.

The adrenal cortex produces several different hormones including the following:

- **Aldosterone:** regulates water and sodium levels, and therefore also plays a crucial role in blood pressure.

- **Cortisol:** involved in the stress response, acts as an anti-inflammatory, and involved in regulating the metabolism.

✄ **Dehydroepiandrosterone (DHEA) & the sulfated form, DHEA-S:** A precursor hormone that converts into multiple important hormones, including testosterone and estradiol.

The adrenal medulla is responsible for the production of catecholamines (norepinephrine and epinephrine/adrenaline), which are responsible for the "fight or flight" response of the sympathetic nervous system.

The function of the adrenal glands is to aid the body in fighting stress from any source, whether it be from an injury, bad health, work exhaustion, emergency, or relationship problems. In fact, these glands will affect any element that can make you tired.

When these glands are overworked, the body will suffer from a condition called adrenal fatigue or exhaustion. This feeling of intense exhaustion can then be felt in the entire body. Thus, hypoadrenia, better known as adrenal fatigue, is a syndrome that occurs when one's adrenal glands work below the required or 'normal' levels. This is commonly associated with long term or severe stress, but can also be the result of an undetected illness. That is why a doctor may associate tiredness with multiple different diseases before the final diagnosis is made.

Adrenal fatigue happens when your HPA (hypothalamic–

pituitary–adrenal) axis cannot keep up with the stress you experience (the organs, i.e. the hypothalamus, the pituitary gland, and the adrenal glands, together with their interactions, make up the HPA axis). The brain is signaling to the adrenals to stop producing cortisol because it has produced enough already, but the adrenals ignore the brain due to repeated stress. They continue producing cortisol as it's the way our bodies have evolved to deal with stress!

Gradually, the entire HPA axis no longer communicate as it used to as the brain is confused that the adrenals aren't responding to its feedback. The brain has told the pituitary to tell the adrenals that they can stop producing cortisol, but the adrenals keep producing cortisol due to the continuation of stress (more on that below).

Then, our adrenals no longer produce sufficient cortisol. Either the adrenal glands can no longer keep up with the demand of cortisol production, or our brain has given up signaling them to produce cortisol, or both factors are present.

HPA axis dysfunction happens because our physiology hasn't evolved to our modern lifestyles yet. We are structured to handle short-term extreme stress (hunting for food) and then longer periods of rest and relaxation. We are also physiologically designed to keep a balance between our sympathetic (fight or flight) and parasympathetic (rest and digest) nervous systems.

Nowadays, not only are we overworked, sleep-deprived, and in sympathetic nervous system overload, but things like poor food quality and even artificial light late at night can be a form of "stress" by our bodies, and thus, our adrenals will respond appropriately.

The stress that affects our adrenals can be emotional, dietary, inflammatory, or environmental.

Emotional stress can be caused by:

- Death, divorce, family issues, or a bad breakup

- Financial troubles

- Feeling unhappy or unsatisfied at work

- Negative thought patterns

- Trauma from experience or PTSD

Dietary stress can be caused by:

- Not eating enough protein

- Eating infrequently

- Eating too many carbohydrates in one sitting

- Other blood sugar imbalances

Inflammatory stress can be caused by:

- An intestinal parasite (often undetected)

- Eating too many inflammatory foods (sugar & processed foods)

- Chronic pain due to inflammation and/or a previous injury

Environmental stress can be caused by:

- Exposure to environmental toxins/pollution

- Sleep deprivation

- Over-working

- Lack of exercise

- Over exercising

Adrenal fatigue can cause destructive behaviors in an individual's life. In severe cases when the adrenal glands' function is greatly diminished, even a menial task such as getting out of bed can be a very difficult task. Every single time there is reduced function of the adrenal glands, the whole-body system is greatly affected.

WHY IT'S HARD TO GET HELP

Adrenal fatigue is still considered a controversial subject, as many individuals still do not consider it to be a real disorder. Although it is becoming more and more common, there are still many doctors who are hesitant or unwilling to give this diagnosis.

There are several reasons for this. The first reason is that lab tests are very inconclusive. For the tests to come back with the correct information, a person's cortisol and DHEA levels would need to be tested several times throughout the day due to the constant fluctuations during a 24-hour period.

The second reason this diagnosis is not more commonly given out is because most of the time, doctors are discouraged from giving it due to both commercial pressures, as well as insurance companies.

When it comes to insurance companies, every disease has its own code. They are known as the International Classification of Disease codes. These are given out by the World Health Organization, which has yet to have a code for Adrenal Fatigue, most likely because all the labs that doctors have been using to try to diagnose it comes back inconclusive.

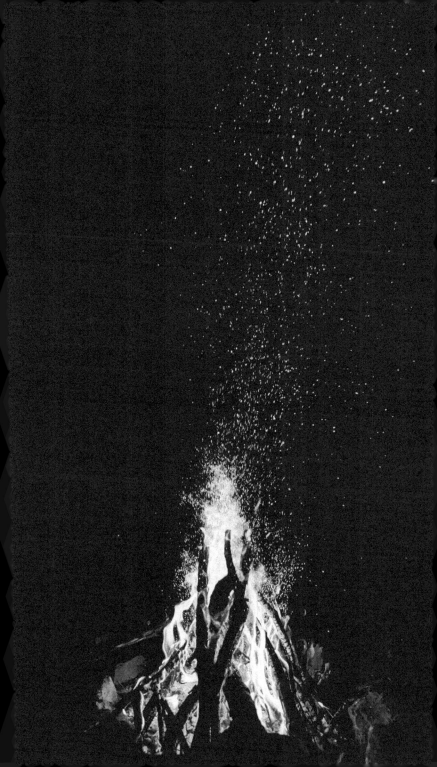

How Adrenals Control Weight, Stress, and Mood

Weight

Weight management is one of the most difficult challenges for many people these days. In fact, obesity is one of the most prevalent conditions in the Western World which puts you at risk for a whole host of issues including heart disease, diabetes, joint degradation, musculoskeletal issues, increased body burden of environmental toxins (fat stores toxins), and shortened life expectancy. It is indeed healthy and even recommended to lose weight if you are carrying around a few extra pounds, especially in the midsection.

Weight Around the Abdomen

Weight-gain around the abdomen is one of the classic signs of adrenal gland dysfunction. When you ask your body to continually release cortisol through an unregulated adrenal response, you are triggering one of the main functions of cortisol: re-depositing fat from the peripheral tissues to the abdominal area. Cortisol mobilizes triglycerides from storage and deposits them into the visceral adipocytes (fat cells). Visceral fat is under the muscle, deep in the abdomen. The primary goal of this is for "organ protection." The problem is, this type of fat is not good for long-term health. In fact, visceral fat increases your predisposition to conditions such as heart disease and diabetes (notice the running theme here).

Cortisol also increases the maturation rate of adipocytes through enzyme control, which converts cortisone into cortisol, via the 11-beta hydroxysteroid dehydrogenase enzyme. Strangely, cortisol regulates its own production by increasing the amount of cortisone being converted to cortisol by stimulating that enzyme. Visceral fat not only has more receptors for cortisol, which means there is greater utilization of cortisol, but also potentially have more of the enzyme to convert cortisone to cortisol.

No wonder it's so hard to lose that weight! It can be extremely hard, but not impossible. In fact, commitment to regular cardiovascular exercise is one of the best ways to shed abdominal fat. The next best thing to do is to get a better handle on your stress response and use strategies such as diet, herbs, and natural therapies to support the adrenal glands and improve lipolysis (breakdown of fat). By incorporating these basic approaches into your daily lifestyle, you will see that the stubborn abdominal fat gradually sheds away.

As a highlight, many people struggle with weight

challenges. Often, weight loss can be challenging for various reasons, including poor dietary choices, yo-yo dieting, and lack of a regular exercise routine. Other major factors affecting your ability to lose weight are your cortisol levels and your stress response. Elevated cortisol causes fat storage and cuts off fuel burning. Therefore, if you struggle with weight loss, make sure your adrenal glands have the right support to get the results you really want.

Stress

Depressed adrenal function is better known as adrenal fatigue or hypoadrenia. It has become one of the major factors affecting health in the modern world. Adrenal fatigue begins when your body responds to acute stressful situations which transitions into a heightened stress response that is maintained by routine stress. When the on-going stress eventually becomes a daily burden, this eventually leads to a depressed adrenal response.

Reaching adrenal fatigue is most common when nothing has been done to keep the adrenal glands healthy or to restore appropriate balance when the function has been compromised. Adrenal fatigue doesn't happen in just one day; it is a process that takes time and develops over years of living a life where your adrenal response is altered and dysfunctional. It is similar to driving your car around without getting the oil changed: eventually you start burning oil, and at some point, you may even damage the engine. Your adrenal glands need regular tune-ups, preferably daily.

The endocrine system, specifically the adrenal glands, works to make sure the organism is reactive and adaptive. The two key words to remember in understanding adrenal gland function, stress, the stress response, and adrenal fatigue is reactive and adaptive. When the body is appropriately reactive and adaptive, it means you can react to stressors and adapt accordingly, then come back into balance after a relatively short amount of time.

Stress is a normal, healthy response to a trigger. Cortisol is essential to life and has numerous biological roles in supporting a healthy body. It is only during stress that the release of cortisol is constant and chronic that symptoms of adrenal fatigue begin.

While it is easy to say that cortisol (produced by the cortex of the adrenal gland) just regulates stress and the stress response, it performs many other balancing activities in the body. You need to think of cortisol first as a health-promoting hormone for this reason: if you didn't have hormones, and didn't have cortisol, you wouldn't be alive. Hormones are extremely important, yet it isn't as easy to just say, "I will remove stress from my life." The way you respond to stressful situations is habitual, so you need to learn how to change your habits. In an effort to understand how you can change your habits, part of the treatment involves mindfulness practices, such as meditation and yoga as it helps to restore balance to your body in stressful situations. Remember: it isn't the stressor but rather your response to it that is affecting your health.

Moods

Are you aware that the adrenal glands constantly produce more than 50 different hormones? If these glands do not function well, one can experience fatigue, mood swings, and other symptoms that result from adrenals attacked by toxins.

The exhaustion caused by Adrenal Fatigue can lead to some changes in mood. Since it's harder for you to stay alert, you may find you're less able to handle stress, become anxious more easily, or are more irritable. It may even seem harder to complete routine work, and self-motivation often becomes an impossible feat.

Many have heard of the saying that "laughter is the best medicine". Well, it's true, especially when it comes to stress! Watching a funny movie, hanging out with friends you can laugh with, or even reading jokes in a magazine can all help to reduce stress. The more you laugh, the better you will cope with the stresses in your life. Try watching the latest family-friendly comedy and enjoy it with the rest of the family!

Laughter releases endorphins in the brain elevating mood and consequently help you deal with stress better. This means your adrenals don't have to work as hard, so laugh loud, laugh long, and laugh often!

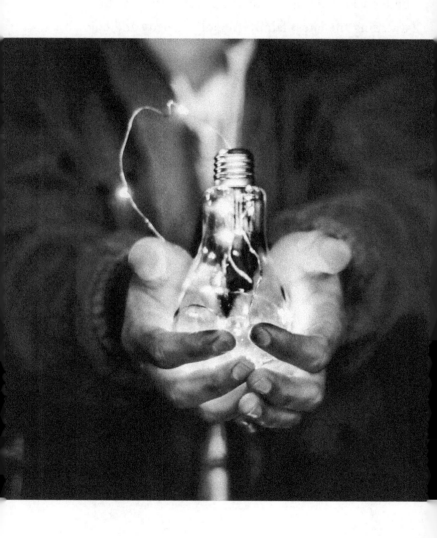

Neurotransmitters and Their Functions

Neurotransmitters are chemicals that transport messages to and from the body to the brain cells. They are responsible for regulating our emotions, behavior, sleep patterns, and learning ability. When your neurotransmitters are in disarray, it causes an imbalance in your body which can lead to an inability to focus or feel good. They influence a person's mood, and are oftentimes linked to mental illnesses and emotional disorders.

They work by transmitting information from neurons to other cells. They are protein in nature since they are made up of amino acids. People should be aware that an imbalance in neurotransmitters can lead to improper functioning of the body's communication system. When one suffers from neurotransmitter imbalances, they are prone to obesity, depression, anxiety, migraines, and ADHD. Other symptoms of neurotransmitter imbalances include bipolar disorders, weight issues, memory impairment, insomnia, fibromyalgia, and hormone and adrenal dysfunction.

Your brain uses neurotransmitters to send messages and trigger reactions by a kind of electrical transmission. Imagine a long queue of people that stretches for miles. If someone at one end of the line wanted to get a message to the person at the other end, they would have one choice – Chinese whispers! That is how your brain communicates except that instead of people, you have individual neurons (brain cells) and instead of a whisper, each neuron releases a certain type of neurotransmitter to get the message across to the other neuron.

There is a gap between each neuron known as a synapse (or the synaptic cleft) and neurotransmitters are your brain's way of getting the message across the gap. The neurotransmitters are stored in vesicles (think of vesicles like little pouches) on the pre-synaptic neuron (the neuron sending the message is known as the pre-synaptic neuron and the neuron receiving the message is, the post-synaptic neuron).

Think of your neurotransmitters as keys which are then needed to open the right locks on the post-synaptic neuron. These locks are known as receptors. When a neurotransmitter fixes to the receptor, it triggers a reaction which cascades through your nervous system using the system likened to the Chinese whispers system mentioned earlier.

If you can imagine a chain of neurons, it is easy to provide a simplified visualization. Imagine the first neuron in the chain. It sends out a message using, say, serotonin, via an axon (imagine a squid with tentacles – the axon is a tentacle that sends messages to nearby neurons). The serotonin will then bind to a specific receptor (called the 5-ht receptor) on a tentacle on the receiving neuron called a dendrite. Axons send the message and dendrites receive.

There are a multitude of neurotransmitters and they are generally classified as either excitatory or inhibitory. This doesn't necessarily mean that they make you "excited" (although neurotransmitters such as norepinephrine and dopamine certainly can), but it just means that they increase the chances that the neuron will go on to fire an action potential. It suffices to say that when a neurotransmitter binds to a receptor, it is no guarantee of a predictable reaction, but a "potential" reaction. The key is for the neurochemical messenger received by the neuron to surpass a threshold of electrical activity. If it does, an action potential will be triggered and if not, it won't.

The main excitatory neurotransmitters are glutamate, acetylcholine, and norepinephrine (and epinephrine), while the primary inhibitory neurotransmitters are GABA, endorphin, and serotonin. Serotonin is complicated and is more accurately called a neuromodulator as it can be either excitatory or inhibitory depending on the context.

The most common neurotransmitters in your nervous system are glutamate and GABA.

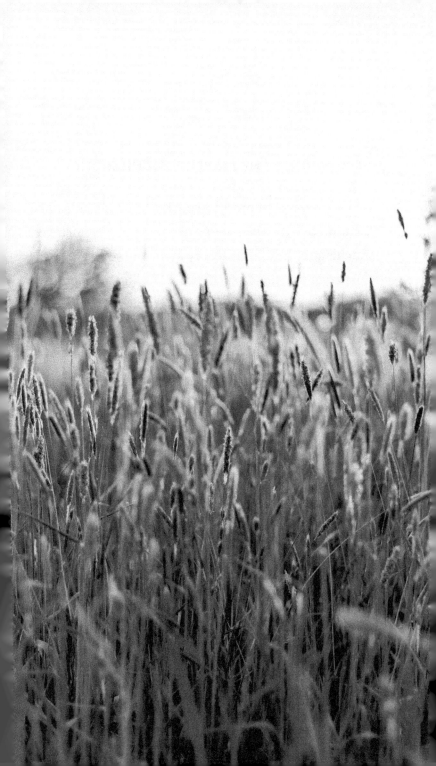

TYPES OF NEUROTRANSMITTERS EXPLAINED

SEROTONIN – THE HAPPINESS ENHANCER

In the evening, some people like to sit outside their homestead with their best friends or family members watching the beautiful scenery of the sun setting. During this moment, they experience a feeling of happiness within and a sense of blessing. This feeling is triggered by the happiness enhancing molecule that is referred to as serotonin. Serotonin is a much desired neurotransmitter in the body since it enhances an optimistic mood.

However, it can be dangerous when there is an imbalance or shortage of serotonin in the brain. Such a situation may end up with feelings of unhappiness, depression, and discontentment in life. Symptoms of serotonin imbalance can present itself differently in men and women. For instance, a man may start being impulsive and result in alcohol abuse, while a woman may be faced with abrupt mood disorders and a craving for carbohydrates.

Excess serotonin can lead to overactive nerve cells, resulting in a fatal collection of symptoms known as Serotonin Syndrome. In most cases, Serotonin

Syndrome symptoms begin within hours of taking a new medication that alters serotonin levels. Some Serotonin Syndrome symptoms include diarrhea, headache, heavy sweating, rapid heart rate, restlessness, agitation, shivers, and changes in blood pressure. In severe cases, symptoms can range from a high fever to seizures.

Working Principle

Serotonin undergoes synthesis and storage before being released into the serotonin pathway by the neurons. Serotonin pathway is the nerve pathway that is mainly influenced by a state of happiness. The function of serotonin depends on the areas it can reach within the brain and the receptors that are meant to receive it. Serotonin plays a crucial role in regulating other brain processes like anxiety, sleep, perception, appetite, aggression, memory, emotion, and mood.

Functions of Serotonin

Serotonin enhances the mood of a person. The neurotransmitter stimulates the brain, making a person active and happy.

When there is an increased amount of serotonin, one starts to experience nausea. This feeling of dizziness needs to be controlled to avoid extreme conditions.

Effects of Serotonin

⚜ Serotonin boosts both the mood and mental health of a person. It improves the happiness of a person, making them elated, and such feelings always have a positive impact to the mental health.

⚜ Serotonin helps in helping us feel lively and builds self-confidence. It is known fact that, when you are happy, you will feel lively and this makes you more attentive and focused in life.

⚜ Serotonin changes in the brain regulate the sleep cycle. The changes and imbalances in serotonin levels are the reason why one is awake during the day and sleeping once it is night.

How to Improve Serotonin Performance?

⚜ Supplemental – 5-HTP, an abbreviation for 5-hydroxytryptophan, is an amino acid that acts as a building block of serotonin. Serotonin is a neurotransmitter found in the human brain. A drop in the quantity of this chemical can provoke anxiety, obesity, and depression, as well as muscular aches and pains. This substance is manufactured naturally by the human body. In some cases, the body does not always make enough. In these cases, a 5-HTP supplements the quantity produced by the body and helps normalize the level of serotonin. Consult your physician before using 5HTP supplements.

- Always expose your body to natural daylight as this will enhance serotonin levels and lowers the risk of depression- and some other disorders that are seasonal.

- Ensure that you work out as it can stimulate your body and enhance the functioning of serotonin within the brain. Exercise increases the serotonin's antidepressant effect.

- Food – the main and most important thing is diet. Neurotransmitters are complicated chemicals and the body needs many building blocks to grow and compensate. Therefore, it is crucial that you have a good balance of protein, vegetables, fruit, and complex carbohydrates to help ensure that you're getting the right building blocks. Also, make sure that you're getting enough Omega 3 essential fatty acids in your diet. Omega 3s are brain foods that boost healthy brain function, and have been demonstrated to be lacking in most diets. Eat foods with a high concentration of tryptophan (like beef, green tea, avocados, chicken and eggs), which is effective in boosting your cognition and mood.

Dopamine

Considering how important dopamine is, our knowledge of what it does exactly in our brains is surprisingly incomplete. As you may have read, dopamine is a catecholamine neurotransmitter, which, along with noradrenaline and glutamate, is one of your main excitatory neurotransmitters.

You have probably read that dopamine is your "pleasure", "motivation", and "reward" neurotransmitter and that, when your brain releases dopamine, it feels great. However,, the reality is a little more complicated.

Our understanding is that when you obtain something important, (from an evolutionary perspective) such as food or sexual gratification, your brain releases a pleasurable rush of dopamine to make you feel "good" and thereby encourages you to repeat the activity. This is why addictive disorders have always been associated with dopaminergic dysfunction, causing people to seek out the same specific thing (such as a drug) over and over. This is considered a dysfunction because it is not hard to imagine the problems that addictive disorders would have created for our distant ancestors.

However, recent research published in the journal Neuron casts some doubt over this simplified understanding. The

Joint Spanish and American study found that it is also dopamine that drives you to seek out these rewards in the first place. Not only that, they also discovered that persistence is likely linked to high dopamine, so the higher the dopamine levels, the more likely you are to soldier on through adversity to achieve a particular goal.

One of the most interesting aspects of dopamine, however, is how it mediates both psychological motivation (towards a goal or reward) and the actual physical movement which carries you towards whatever the goal happens to be. The part of the brain that is responsible for this, the basal ganglia, is largely controlled by dopamine. If you look at a glass of water and decide to pick it up and drink it because you are thirsty, it is dopamine (via the basal ganglia) which controls the initiation of movement which brings your hand to the glass to pick it up. Therefore, when the dopamine-producing neurons in a part of the basal ganglia known as the substantia nigra are destroyed, Parkinson's disease or other similar disorders are the result.

I bet you thought things couldn't get more complicated regarding dopamine, right? In recent years, the situation has become further clouded by the concept of reward prediction error. Scientists conducting rodent experiments have found that the dopaminergic system is much more complicated than we thought. The classical understanding of dopamine is that an animal sees food (or a potential mate) and consequently experiences a pleasurable burst of dopamine to encourage it to see the reward and is then motivated to do something similar again in the future.

However, there is a problem with this that you may know from personal experience. Imagine you are walking down the street and you notice an ice cream store has opened. You proceed inside and order the most delicious ice cream you have ever tasted. How good is that feeling? The next time you pass by that ice cream store, you will get a little jolt of dopaminergic pleasure thinking about getting one of those great ice creams again. We all know how this story ends. By the fifth or tenth time (or sooner in some cases), you have grown accustomed to getting that ice cream and you no longer get much pleasure from it. In fact, if you check your state of mind closely, you may find that you thought you were getting pleasure but was just really chasing a kind of ephemeral pleasure and was simply acting out of habit.

Unfortunately, dopamine is a "MORE MORE MORE!" neurotransmitter and is never happy with the same thing over and over. You feel the need to keep chasing that bigger and better pleasure. Dopamine loves novelty, which is why travel can give us so much pleasure. To put it in another way, if something (like ice cream) is abundant, the parts of your brain responsible for reward and reinforcement (which use dopamine to signal) lose interest, as they assume that they don't need to ensure you to take advantage of it since it isn't as rare as the first few times.

This understanding underpins the concept of reward prediction error and has thrown up interesting results in animal trials. Researchers found that when a mouse experienced the same reward more than once, dopamine wasn't just automatically released when the mouse saw the reward again. Dopamine levels only rose if the reward was greater than expected and if the reward was less than expected, dopamine levels dropped.

So, in summary, dopamine likes new experiences, rare things and pleasant surprises.

The parts of the brain which are mainly managed by dopamine are the basal ganglia (which you already know about), the nucleus accumbens (which is part of the basal ganglia, to be specific) and the ventral tegmental area (VTA). I want to avoid focusing on individual brain structures too much because this is not a neurology book. Besides that, when we look at structures of the brain, we can disappear down a rabbit hole that doesn't get us any closer to understanding how our minds work.

However, in some cases, specific mention of particular brain structures can be instructive.

What are the symptoms of low dopamine?

The symptoms of low dopamine are generally unsurprising when you think of it as your energy/mood/pleasure neurotransmitter. However, there are one or two symptoms which are less obvious:

- Hypersomnia (too much sleep) and difficulty getting out of bed in the morning.

- Lack of ability to feel pleasure from the things that normally interest you (anhedonia). It is also difficult to clearly differentiate between "pleasure" and "happiness". Can you tell the difference? This is one of the reasons why people sometimes get confused when they hear both serotonin and dopamine referred to as "the feel-good neurotransmitter". In general, serotonin is a more contented, relaxed kind of positive mood whereas dopamine is a more excited, motivated and (sometimes) euphoric kind of positive mood.

- Lack of motivation

- Low motivation/lack of pleasure/apathetic depression.

- More introverted than usual.

- Lack of mental energy.

- Addictive personality related to your reward and pleasure center (your nucleus accumbens in particular) involving things such as drugs or sex.

- Reduced sex drive

Gamma Amino Butyric Acid (GABA)

GABA is your brain's most important inhibitory neurotransmitter. Glutamate puts the foot on the accelerator and GABA is the brake. If you are like most people, you would have felt the effects of GABA at least once or twice – benzodiazepine sedatives (or benzos, as they are commonly referred to) like Xanax and Valium work by boosting the activity of GABA, leading to reduced anxiety and, eventually, sleep.

This is why this class of drug is the most potent treatment (excluding barbiturates, which I won't get started on…) for anxiety possible. If you boost GABA levels enough, it is virtually impossible to feel anxious.

However, GABA is associated with the same problems (and more) as dopamine – boosting GABA quickly develops tolerance and then leads to addictive behavior.

Some people believe benzos to be as addictive as heroin. There is also another important downside to boosting GABA with drugs like benzos – they tend to be neurotoxic in higher doses for extended periods of time. If you ever saw someone who had abused benzos for a long time, you would be shocked. These people are completely fried. This is not a path you want to go down.

Probably the only non-neurotoxic way I know to boost GABA is via anti-convulsive medications like gabapentin (Neurontin) and pregabalin (Lyrica). In fact, because these drugs can prevent glutamate toxicity (where glutamate levels are overactive, damaging neurons), there is an argument to suggest that for some people, they are neuroprotective. The key seems to be that these types of drugs don't boost GABA directly; they actually boost GABA by suppressing glutamate. To use the car analogy again, benzos put the foot hard on the brake, whereas drugs like Lyrica slow the car by taking the foot off the accelerator.

Other ways include consuming foods that have a high concentration of glutamates like oranges, oats, almonds, potato, beef liver, bananas, whole wheat, lentils, and spinach. Also, practice yoga 3 to 4 times a week.

Lastly, you may have seen GABA supplements for sale in a health food store. Don't bother. There is very little evidence that oral GABA crosses the blood-brain barrier in any meaningful amount. GABA is like glutathione in that way – you are better off fixing it indirectly.

ENDORPHIN

It is also called the endogenous morphine. Its key role is to calm down an individual by reducing their stress and pain. If there is an insufficient amount within the brain, it can result in psychiatric and eating disorders.

How it works:

They work by transmitting electrical signals between various parts of the nervous system, especially the pituitary glands found in the human brain. Endorphins are triggered by the presence of pain and stress, thereby communicating with opiate receptors that help in reducing pain sensitivity.

Functions of Endorphins:

- They aid in the release of energy into the brain to produce a sense of relaxation after a workout.

- They help in reducing or eliminating pain

- They improve a person's mood, making them happier.

How to Improve Performance:

- You need to laugh often to encourage the release of endorphins and that will help reduce stress to a manageable level.

- Play good music to improve your mood and, hence, the release of more endorphins.

- Inhale the aromas from vanilla or lavender. Your anxiety will be lowered and your mood will be enhanced.

- Always exercise, which leads to good health and the release of endorphins.

NOREPINEPHRINE

It is also referred to as an excitatory neurotransmitter. It plays a role in enhancing the memory of individuals, helping them to remember events and activities done on a daily basis. It works by keeping your body active and energetic by increasing your heart rate and taking control of your glucose level and blood pressure.

Symptoms of low Norepinephrine include depression, anxiety, decreased focus levels, inconsistent sleeping cycles, bad moods, and low energy. You simply need to workout consistently to get rid of such conditions.

Norepinephrine's Functions:

✂ Norepinephrine works by shutting down metabolic processes like growth, energy vitalization, digestion, and flow of blood. This gives the brain ample time to understand such processes to improve its performance.

✂ Oxygen flow is improved since norepinephrine will increase your breathing rate. This implies that your brain functioning is improved due to adequate oxygen supply.

✂ Norepinephrine contributes to the release of increased amounts of glucose, thus increasing the strength of your muscle.

How to Improve Performance:

✂ Eat foods that are rich in tyrosine like seafood, oatmeal, meat, fish, chicken, bananas, cheese, chocolate, and chicken.

✂ You may use supplements as well. These include Acetyl-l- tyrosine that enhances your memory and Arctic root to boost your energy. Always get advice from your doctor before using them.

✂ Take cold showers and have a good exercise routine.

⚜ Always have daytime naps which relaxes your brain and increase norepinephrine levels.

Epinephrine

Its function is to aid in controlling attention, cognition, arousal, and even mental focus. It is an excitatory neurotransmitter that regulates our metabolic rate.

Symptoms for absence of epinephrine include high blood pressure, increased heart rate, insomnia, and prolonged stress. The absence can lead to problems of the heart, as well as behavioral and mental disorders.

Epinephrine's working principle includes muscle relaxation, regulation of metabolic rate, and constriction of blood vessels found in the brain.

Epinephrine's Functions:

⚜ The neurotransmitter helps an individual to adequately respond to fear by fighting it. When there is fear, epinephrine is released, making the brain release signals which caution against danger and a response of fighting back.

⚜ It improves your attentiveness, focus, and concentration.

How to Improve Performance:

- ✂ Ensure enough rest to increase the release of adrenaline.

- ✂ Always work to meet deadlines to avoid the consequences of incomplete tasks, learn how to manage your time efficiently.

- ✂ Stay conscious of your surroundings to improve your awareness of events and objects around you.

GLUTAMATE

Glutamate is an excitatory neurotransmitter that enhances our memory and learning process through what we face daily. The neurotransmitter is located in the brain's central nervous system and strengthens an individual's memorizing and learning capabilities. Excess glutamate can lead to Lou Gehrig's disease - amyotrophic lateral sclerosis (ALS). This can be in the form of brain damage or a stroke and can result in death.

Glutamate's Functions:

- ✂ It helps the memory to function in terms of learning and memory capabilities.

- ✂ It enhances the level of concentration in an individual and enhancing memory.

Glutamate's Effects:

- ❉ It enhances an individual's concentration and focus. Such a person will have a high thinking capacity.

- ❉ Focus and good memory improves intelligence, which is brought about by excessive amounts of glutamate.

How to Improve Performance:

- ❉ Always find time to workout. This helps the nerve cells in the brain to multiply and strengthen. This results in improved learning and cognition functions.

- ❉ Use supplements that consists of cinnamon, coconut milk, whey milk and berries to boost the glutamate's level.

- ❉ A nice sleep cycle balances the glutamate levels within the brain.

ACETYLCHOLINE

This is a neurotransmitter that functions as a learning and memory enhancing molecule. A deficit has grave consequences such Alzheimer's. During the sleep cycle, this neurotransmitter causes rapid eye movement (REM).

Acetylcholine, like glutamate, is a key neurotransmitter for controlling aspects of arousal and attention, although in a slightly different way. Acetylcholine is distributed all throughout your body and brain, where it controls a range of functions such as muscle control and reward behavior. Acetylcholine is possibly the prototypical neurotransmitter in the classic understanding of a substance that is used to send messages from one part of the brain to another, or to the peripheral nervous system. For example, if you decide to pick up a glass of water, there will be a long chain of acetylcholine signaling. The releases of acetylcholine is followed by the binding of the receptors, which triggers more release and so on, down the chain, until it results in a muscular contraction that enable you to pick up that glass of water.

Acetylcholine's Working Principle:

Acetylcholine stimulates the brain's muscles by ensuring that they contract from time to time, which in turn relaxes the muscles of the heart. It affects the arousal effect and learning capacity that are regulated by the central nervous system.

Acetylcholine's Functions:

Acetylcholine serves as an activator and an inhibitor at the same time. It sends and receives messages within the brain as well as facilitating muscle movement, making it easier for the body to detect pain.

How to Improve Performance:

Eat foods that are rich in choline such as poultry, dairy, fish, meat, broccoli, whole wheat, Brussel sprouts, and peanut butter.

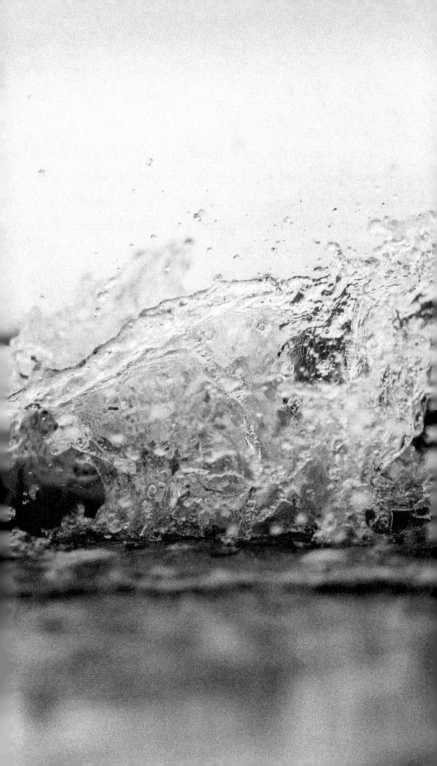

Neurotransmitters and Adrenal Fatigue are Connected

There are two adrenal glands in our body. They are both positioned on top of the kidneys. These glands are responsible for the production of important endorphins, together with noradrenaline and adrenaline, and assist the body in managing stress.

When the body is undergoing chronic stress, the neurotransmitter epinephrine (also known as adrenaline) is secreted in a continuous manner and your body maintains a state of flight or fight. The adrenals will respond to this situation by producing the stress hormone cortisol to deal with the threat you are currently facing. This will result in increased focus, blood pressure, heart rate, and decision-making. The presence of cortisol will slow down system functions of the body that are not pertinent for survival like the immune, reproductive, and digestive systems.

Why is such a situation important? When there is a threat to your survival, the *flight or fight* response will make your senses hyperalert and the brain is tasked to think critically so that it can assess the best solution to the situation to either attack, escape, or survive with the danger. This can be an immense help to individuals, giving them a chance to avoid and survive any unpredictable dangers, cases of financial problems, relationships hitting rocks, and even when one runs late for a scheduled appointment.

Such a response is commonly known as the NeuroEndoMetabolic (NEM) Stress Response. This is the natural way the body defends itself against stress. Upon the release of cortisol, the systems of the body are affected in a negative way. Excessive NEM Stress Response due to chronic stress results in adrenal fatigue.

Multiple studies have been carried out to establish the relationship between adrenal fatigue and neurotransmitters. It has been established that an imbalance of serotonin and dopamine may result in illnesses such as fibromyalgia and chronic fatigue syndrome. Neurotransmitters cause the body to stimulate the adrenal glands to increase the production of stress-fighting hormones.

Eventually, your adrenals cannot generate enough from the body's hormones that you might want. Because of this, your own levels of cortisol, in addition to neurotransmitters, as is the case of adrenaline in addition to norepinephrine, are usually lesser than they should be. Adrenal Fatigue is caused when there is an imbalance of neurotransmitters, for instance the lack of serotonin and GABA.

The neurotransmitter acetylcholine, adrenal fatigue and thiamine deficiency connection.

The classification of neurons is based on the neurotransmitter they make use of. You will find that adrenergic nerve fibers utilizes epinephrine and/or norepinephrine while cholinergic nerve fibers use acetylcholine. The adrenergic neurons are termed as stimulatory while cholinergic nerves fibers are inhibitory. In relation to the autonomic nervous system, the parasympathetic branch has cholinergic nerve fibers while the sympathetic nervous system has adrenergic nerve fibers.

The autonomic nervous system has two branches aimed at promoting the survival of an organism. The two branches include the sympathetic and parasympathetic. The sympathetic nervous system gets your body ready for flight or fight by initiating a stress response to get the needed resources for the situation. The parasympathetic branch is responsible for the recovery process from stress.

The vagus nerve is the passage through which the brain and the gut communicate and functions to control the parasympathetic branch. The vagus nerve fibers are purported to be cholinergic (thus using acetylcholine as its main neurotransmitter). Acetylcholine is responsible for contraction of muscles. It is also one of the main neurotransmitters in the parasympathetic nervous system. It was discovered that it is involved in the neural circuit called the inflammatory reflex. You should note that the inflammatory reflex connects the nervous and immune systems, in which case the nervous system regulates the process of inflammation. The vagus nerves are stimulated by inflammatory cytokines and signal the brain, which then delivers a message to the celiac ganglion (the meeting point of parasympathetic nerve fibers and sympathetic fibers). The spleen releases T cells after it is triggered by the sympathetic fibers. This action leads to the production of acetylcholine, which reduces the inflammation.

Optimal synthesis of acetylcholine within the neurons depends on reliable glycolysis. Acetyl CoA and choline are synthesized to form Acetylcholine. Acetyl CoA originates from glycolysis as triglycerides cannot be metabolized by nerves. While some Acetyl CoA is synthesized from acetate, others incorporated in acetylcholine is sourced from pyruvate (because of glycolysis).

Adequate thiamine is needed by neurons for pyruvate to be converted to Acetyl CoA. For the processes that need acetylcholine, thiamine plays a very big role.

Do the aforementioned details link to adrenal fatigue? It should be noted that constant inflammation increases acetylcholine requirements because of the inflammatory reflex trigger. This is determined by the presence of Acetyl CoA and choline. Constant inflammation in neurons causes thiamine deficiency in two ways. The first way is where GI inflammation interferes with the uptake of thiamine into your bloodstream. The second way is when thiamine needs are above the required levels due to increased acetylcholine.

For those who suffer from Type 2 diabetes, experiencing this state of chronic inflammation is considered the norm. In addition, thiamine metabolism and status are poorly modulated, which may result in chronic inflammation. Such individuals experience low levels of vagus nerve function and a high chronic sympathetic tone. This implies that they are constantly in a state of stress or, what we refer to as adrenal fatigue. Thus, the deficiency of thiamine has negative impacts on adrenal function.

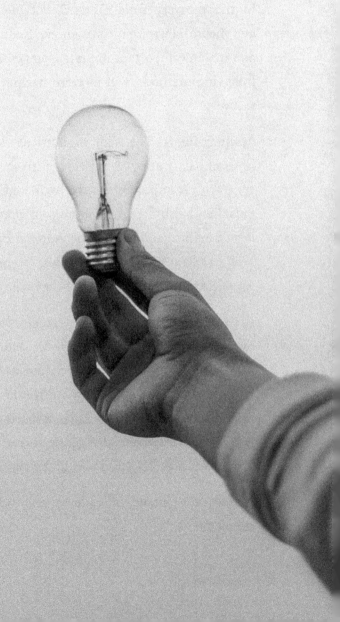

REGAINING BALANCE

✓ Restoring balance to the body and mind is essential in the recovery from Adrenal Fatigue Syndrome and neurotransmitter imbalances. Reducing stress and making important lifestyle changes, such as the following methods, will increase healing and speed recovery.

✓ Maintaining a diet high in nutrient dense foods is essential. Eating a variety of fresh fruits and vegetables is important for the brain and body. Lean meats and fish are great sources of protein, as are beans, quinoa, and lentils. The Adrenal Fatigue Diet is an excellent model that provides optimal nutrition for rejuvenation and healing of the body.

✓ A neurotransmitter imbalance can also be improved by Tai chi. Exercise is key to achieving and maintaining optimal health. Sufferers of Adrenal Fatigue Syndrome and neurotransmitter imbalances may find exercise difficult. It is important to begin with minimal impact and gentle forms of physical activity, such as Yoga, Tai Chi, and walking.

✓ Reduce the intake of caffeine and other energy supplements.

✓ Limit the consumption of alcohol.

✓ Use vitamin and mineral supplements as directed. Individuals with Adrenal Fatigue Syndrome and an imbalance of neurotransmitters should use caution and consult their medical professional about the use of supplements. Some supplements, such as 5-htp and Glutamine, may have an unintended response or paradoxical reaction.

✓ Sleep is vital! Practice good sleep hygiene, such as maintaining regular sleep and wake times, using the bed only for sleep and sex (no reading or electronics in bed), and limiting caffeine and energy supplements at least six hours before bedtime.

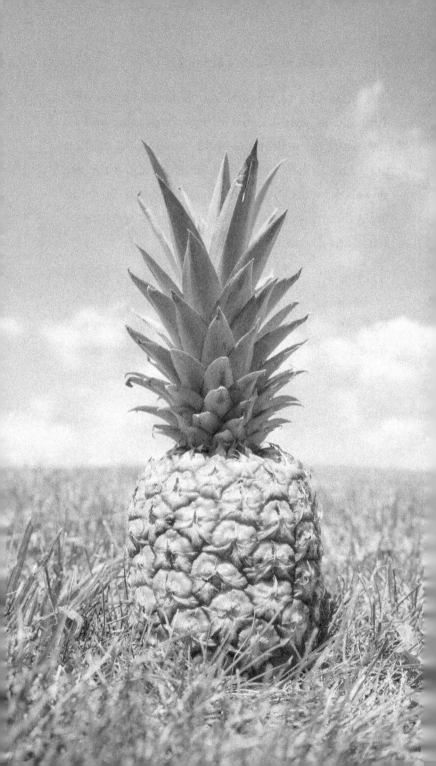

Regaining Your Energy

Fatigue is terrible! Fatigue is much more than just tiredness. Some people suffering from adrenal fatigue find it impossible to make it through an entire day without becoming overwhelmingly exhausted to the point where they must lie down and rest.

Fatigue can impact your everyday life in all aspects. You might be late to work because you miss your alarm every morning or your decision making is at its worst in the middle of the day.

You may even have started losing friends because you can't seem to get out of bed to socialize on your time off. You also most likely have lost interest in your favorite hobbies because you simply don't have the energy for them anymore.

The most important thing that you want to focus on when you're suffering from adrenal fatigue is getting your energy back. As mentioned, diet is your first line of defense against adrenal fatigue. When you're experiencing chronic fatigue, it is absolutely imperative that you follow a diet rich in nutrients and whole foods.

When you eat healthy and natural foods that are low in

(bad) fat and high in vitamins, you're giving your body the fuel and nutrients it needs to repair, recover, and keep on chugging along.

Below, you will read important tips to keep your energy levels up naturally, the best natural foods for boosting energy, and some great recipes to help you recover from adrenal fatigue and keep you going all day long.

First, Rule Out Medical Problems!

Check with your doctor to evaluate the cause and follow the advice you receive. It is quite possible that your doctor will want you to go through an examination and have blood tests to rule out other probable causes and confirm the diagnosis. This is then followed up with treatment.

Eat Throughout Day

The best favor you can do for your body is to eat small amounts of food every three to four hours instead of cramming high amounts of calories into two or three large meals.

You ought to eat at regular intervals throughout the day as it will provide you with all the right nutrients and vitamins you require to stay energized all day long. Not only is this helpful for boosting energy, it also regulates your metabolism and hormones, which help you curb cravings, reduce stress, and lose weight.

Do Not Skip Breakfast

There is so much truth to the sentence that we have all heard about a billion times before: breakfast is the most vital meal of the day! Breakfast gives you the energy you need to start your day. It boosts your metabolism and kick-starts your brain. If you want to heal your body, get more energy, lose weight, and stay healthy, you should definitely have your breakfast at the start of each day.

If you constantly feel fatigue, it can seem like an impossible feat to drag yourself out of bed early enough to eat a healthy meal before you begin taking care of business. However, for the sake of your own mental and physical well-being, you must eat breakfast! You'll be surprised to see how much it helps you to feel energized after you start eating it regularly.

Start an Exercise Routine

It may not be the easy but once you've started doing something physically, the energy you experience will go back to normal levels. Remember that energy creates energy. A journey of a thousand miles begin with a single step!

Drink Water

This is one of the main reasons individuals feel weak - they are simply dehydrated!

Go to Bed Early

Sleeping late affects the body in so many ways and can be the cause of your fatigue.

Stress Control

Talk to a friend, a family member, a psychologist, or anyone you can trust. Letting it all out will lessen the burden and help you to overcome the fatigue. If you don't want to weigh down a friend, a professional may be a better choice.

Reduce Work Load

Overworking certainly can cause adrenal fatigue, so try slowing down and take breaks often if possible.

Avoid Caffeine

Before we begin with our list of natural and healthy energy boosting recipes and meal plans, we preface the remainder of this chapter with this very important word of advice. If you have been diagnosed with, or believe you may be suffering from adrenal fatigue, stay away from caffeine!

The energy your body derives from caffeine is short lived. You've surely heard of a caffeine crash, and maybe you've experienced one yourself – that exhausting part of the afternoon, a couple of hours after you've stopped pumping your body full of that morning brew, where you suddenly feel drained of every ounce of energy you had in you and all you want to do is lie down somewhere and take a nap.

Not only does caffeine cause your body and mind to crash, but over time it will have less of an effect on you as well. Your body starts building up tolerance to it and you will need more caffeine to have the same effect on you. Stimulating your body with caffeine all the time also weakens your adrenal glands, which obviously does not help you recover from adrenal fatigue. You must avoid caffeine at all costs if you really want to get better.

Limit Alcohol Consumption

Alcohol has a sedative effect which reduces energy levels and would not be helpful for productivity.

Eat More Soluble Fiber

This will even out your energy levels as it prevents blood sugar levels from spiking and eventually crashing.

Supplement with Vitamin C & B

Several studies have shown that there is a correlation between severe fatigue and vitamin C deficiency. Vitamin B also aids in the conversion of blood sugar into energy.

Avoid or Quit Smoking

Nicotine affects your sleeping habits which makes you feel tired and cranky for most of the day.

Listen to Music

This is not just a wives' tale but has been proven that listening to music can help energize the body and help you feel upbeat in no time. In fact, you could even try dancing as this has beneficial therapeutic effects.

Listen to Your Body Clock

Try to understand your body rhythm and adjust to it.

Try Chocolate

This will probably be a relief to you - especially if you're someone who has a sweet tooth. There is an endorphin buzz when you eat chocolate which will boost your energy. This is why explorers use it to increase their energy levels under extreme conditions.

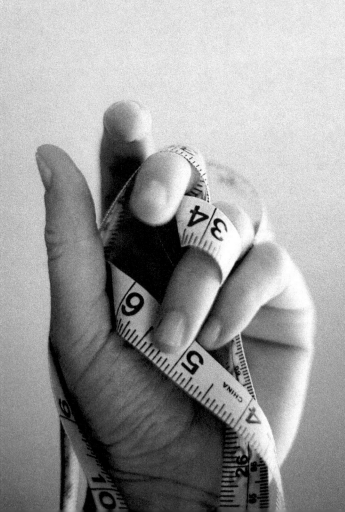

The power of the mind over the body is often overlooked in modern medicine. In recent years, it has been found that psychological changes have a real impact on our physical health. Stress is a fitting example as it is a mental state that has the power to trigger many different physical changes within our bodies. These changes can impact almost all organs or systems that are vital to our health. Prolonged exposure to stress can lead to chronic illnesses such as adrenal fatigue. Hence, one of the ways to improve chronic fatigue syndrome is to address the main causes of stress in our lives. Since our mental health can cause physical problems, it is also assumed that improving our emotional well-being can help reverse these disorders.

Stress Less – if you can't eradicate stress completely from your life, then strive to keep it to a minimum. This is one of the key concepts of the diet because if you are stressed out, your body is more likely to turn and store any food that you consume into fat instead of metabolizing it into energy.

Exercise

Which stage of adrenal fatigue you are in determines what

type of exercises you can safely perform. If you are in the last two stages, your adrenal glands cannot produce the hormones needed for vigorous activities such as going for a run or soccer because, once the temporary high is over, it will inevitably result in an adrenal crash. Low impact exercises such as swimming, yoga, or walking are better. If you are in the first two stages, you can lift weights and go for runs as exercise tends to help regulate cortisol levels.

In the adrenal reset diet, there are three ways to exercise depending on your stress levels. If you are in the first level of stress, in which you have difficulty falling asleep, mentally scattered, or feeling edgy, go for strength training. If you are on the second level of stress where your energy levels are low in the morning, become erratic during the day and being alert at night making it difficult for you to get quality sleep, opt for cardio exercises. Alternate between high and low-intensity cardio exercises. If you are very stressed and you constantly crave salty or sugary sweet foods, waking up from sleep not feeling refreshed, and your energy levels are always low, then go for gentle exercises such as slow-paced yoga or a leisurely walk once in the morning and once in the evening

Start your exercise routine early in the day; waiting too long can disrupt your natural sleep cycles. If you get it done early, you also reap the added benefit of a metabolism boost. People who are older find that prolonged periods of exercise drain too much energy while younger people can exercise for longer periods of time. Be careful not to overexert yourself to the point of exhaustion.

Deep Breathing and Meditation

Studies show that meditation can change our circulatory patterns, brain waves, and immune response. That is impressive considering most of the medical world often forget or neglect the power of the mind over the body. Meditation and deep breathing can be beneficial at all four stages. If you are in the first two stages, it can help you reduce stress and stabilize adrenaline and cortisol levels. If you are in the last two stages, it can help you improve circulation and increase energy levels.

Meditation can sound difficult; it is often very hard for us to sit still for two minutes, which makes 15 or 20 minutes seem nearly impossible. However, there are many reasons to do it, so find a nice quiet area and settle yourself for at least 15 minutes. It is unnecessary to force yourself into the lotus position. If you are uncomfortable that way, you can sit on the floor with your hands on your lap, or you can even sit in a chair. The critical point is to ensure you maintain the natural curve of your back. Gently close your eyes and start by taking slow, deep breaths, inhaling through your nose and exhaling through your mouth. Your first few breaths will most likely be shallow, but as you continue to breathe, they will become full and deep. Focus on each breath you take, be aware of the air entering and exiting your lungs. If you find your attention straying, simply bring it back by letting thoughts float by, try your best to not get frustrated, just continue to focus on your breathing. Practice makes perfect and the more you meditate, the easier it will be to maintain focus. When it is time to end the session, open your eyes and slowly stand up. Repeat this once or twice a day.

Carb Timing

Contrary to popular belief, carbs are not actually the enemy. Eating carbs at the right time, choosing the right carbs, and pairing them with protein-rich foods can help you lose weight. With proper timing and the right carbohydrates, you can also achieve better sleep quality, which in turn helps to lower stress levels. In the adrenal reset diet, carb-rich foods are a big NO. Again, this goes against popular belief, so try to change your mind-set when it comes to breakfast and stock up on protein rich foods. Then, build up carbohydrates slowly from lunch with the largest amounts of carbs for dinner. Carbohydrate rich vegetables are also recommended during meal times or in between meals. Again, carb timing is essential in this diet as this will help you regulate your cortisol back to homeostasis or healthy rhythms. Furthermore, it also promotes good sleep and will help you to be alert throughout the day.

Stress Reduction

There are some things you can do to help yourself deal with stress. This can be done by preparing yourself for the situation ahead. For instance, if you anticipate a business meeting, make sure you have everything ready. You can even lay out your clothes and prepare your breakfast that will keep overnight to allow you more time in the morning.

Listening to meditative or soft music helps to alleviate stress. You can even do this on your way to work. Add some muscle relaxation exercises by holding onto your steering wheel and clench the muscles in your back, arms, shoulders, and fingers until they tremble, hold this for 45 seconds and then release. This will cause a wave of relief to spread throughout your upper body.

A Swedish study found that floating in water can trigger the body's relaxation response, which helps lower stress hormone levels. If you are uncomfortable in the water, then do not attempt this as it may increase your stress levels. Choose activities based on your preferences and limitations.

Learning to worry about one thing at a time can go a long way in helping you cope with stress in a way that is healthy. Doing this keeps you from feeling overwhelmed by having multiple problems looming over you. Learn to identify real-life problems and tune out imagined ones. The brain cannot tell the difference between a real and perceived threat, so imagined stressors can have just as much impact as a real stressor.

Talk or write about what is bothering you. If you have friends or family members that you feel comfortable talking to, set up to meet with them. If that is not an option, writing in a journal or even blogging is enough to make you feel less alone.

Learn to speak a stress-free language, people who handle stress well tend to use what stress specialists refer to as an "optimistic explanatory style." They do not dwell on things that don't work out in their favor, and instead of making negative statements, they would focus on one thing they could do better. Instead of saying you "expect" something, train yourself to say "hope" instead.

Laughter improves immune function and relieves tension, but one of the fastest way to kill a sense of humor is anxiety and stress. With that logic, it would also mean that it is almost impossible to feel stressed when you are in the middle of a laughing fit. So, watch that comedy that never fails to make you laugh or hang out with your funniest friend.

Attempt the impossible and pick out one good thing that happened every day and reflect on it. This is a common scenario for many of us: reaching home and immediately venting to our spouse or roommate about what an awful day it has been. Next time, instead of creating a negative atmosphere, try something positive.

No matter how tired you are, don't skip your workout routine. Make sure you stick to your schedule and avoid skipping workouts because it can become a bad habit. Exercise is one of the best ways to help release stress, but you can only reap this benefit if you make it part of your routine.

Having a positive and open mind is one of your best weapons against adrenal fatigue. As you have learned, the influence of the mind over the body can be powerful, and the same can be said for attitude. You are more likely to succeed if you think positively and are open to making changes. If you go into it with a negative outlook, you will only cause yourself more stress while slowing your progress and recovery. Do not beat yourself up over your mistakes, instead, correct your behavior and continue to move on.

You can do one relaxation or stress relieving technique or combine a few of them to find what works best for you. Meditation is recommended for all who suffer from adrenal fatigue since it has so many benefits, but how you do it is according to your personal preference. Everyone who suffers from adrenal fatigue wishes there was a simple cure that works quickly but recovery takes a lot of work and can take anywhere from 6 to 18 months. However, once you start to make some progress, you will feel re-energized and want to keep making these positive changes. Just keep working towards your goal and continue the stress reduction techniques that works for you and, before you realize it, you will be well on your way to a full recovery.

Recovery depends on various factors such as the severity of the adrenal fatigue and your willingness to make the necessary lifestyle changes. The more severe the adrenal fatigue, the longer it takes to recover. Instead of rushing it, take joy in the little things that make it easier. Celebrate the small breakthroughs. Smaller goals are easier and faster to achieve, and they add up to much larger goals. The path to recovery can be difficult, but with patience and hard work, you can get there.

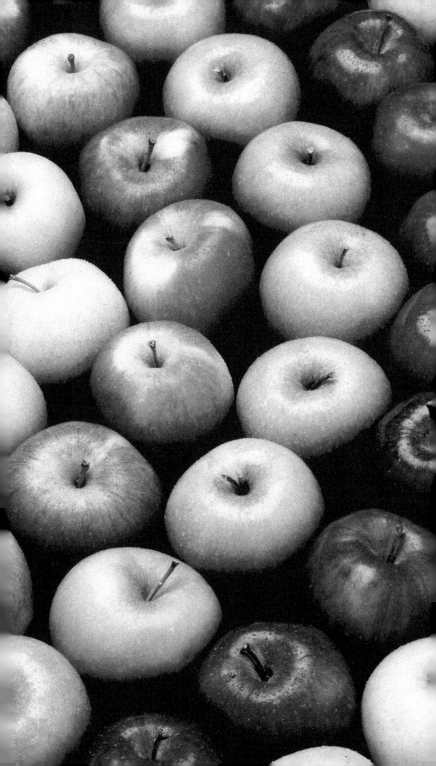

Power Foods for Adrenal Fatigue

Changing your lifestyle and having a proper diet are the first steps towards a healthier lifestyle. Escaping from a stressful life is a dream come true for many people. Though this is not easily achieved, you can reach it through strict control over your own body and what you eat.

Changing your diet and eating the right meals at the right time will give you a healthy mind and a fit body. A healthy body and mind is what many aspire to have yet quite difficult to achieve. It can be accomplished by making changes to your eating habits and it will consequently restore your health. Isn't this enough motivation to start healing yourself?!

So far, you need to have information on the foods you should avoid to improve the functioning of the adrenal glands. Below are some amazing foods that you should include in your diet to improve adrenal function:

Bone broth

The bone broth has been used for centuries for healing purposes due to its nutritional value. Bone marrow is the main component of bone broth. It has been found to have anti-inflammatory properties and can also help in boosting your immune system and in increasing good cholesterol. Bone marrow also provides essential amino acids, minerals, and vitamins, which are essential for optimal functioning of the adrenal glands.

Seaweed

Seaweeds are high in nutrients and minerals that are hard to find in your average diet. These nutrients are important in improving your adrenal function. You can mix the seaweed in salads.

Fermented Drinks

Some fermented drinks are extremely good for your immune system and for the enhancement of your digestive health. This does not necessarily refer to beer, that is unhealthy for you. Fermented drinks such as kvass and kombucha are high in minerals, contain good bacteria, and can greatly improve nutrient absorption and digestion to relieve some load on your adrenals.

Adrenal Reset Dieting Tips

Don't skip breakfast or any other meal - the most important meal of the day is breakfast. Make sure you don't skip it as it kick-starts metabolism and raises your blood sugar, thus keeping you energized throughout the day. Eating breakfast also reduces the chances of eating unhealthy snacks, such as highly processed foods, that can strain your adrenal glands. Ensure you eat your breakfast an hour after waking up.

Do not over eat: Overeating increases the load on your digestive system, which in turn increases the workload of your adrenals and can make you feel tired.

Do not let yourself get too hungry: If you are hungry, instead of waiting for your regular mealtime, eat smaller meals at regular intervals. When you suffer from adrenal fatigue, your body experiences difficulties storing energy. Regular meals are important to replenish your energy levels.

Eat a snack an hour before bed: Eat a healthy snack before you go to bed to energize your body as you sleep so that you don't wake up feeling tired.

Make sure your meals contain protein, fat, and carbs: This enables you to get all the nutrients you need for sufficient energy.

Add some healthy fats to your meals: As mentioned earlier, healthy fats are good for you when suffering from adrenal fatigue. Therefore, make sure you consume healthy fats such as coconut oil, butter, flaxseed oil, and walnut oil.

Avoid white flours and white sugars: These carbohydrates demand a greater release of insulin and cortisol to manage your sugar levels. This increases the stress to your adrenal glands by making it more difficult for them to keep up with the demand for insulin while also stabilizing the levels of your blood sugar. You can choose better alternatives for sugar by using raw honey, palm sugar, or xylitol.

Avoid the intake of alcohol: Drinking alcohol is not good for you when suffering from adrenal fatigue. Alcohol is broken down into simple sugars thus necessitating your body to release insulin and cortisol, which manages the sugar levels in the body. This extra stress on the adrenal glands worsens the situation. Therefore, if you want to get better, you need to avoid alcohol. You can start by reducing your intake with the goal of eventually not consuming alcohol at all.

As you change your diet, it is also important to avoid foods that you may be sensitive or allergic to. Food sensitivities and allergies may only present a while later, after eating the food. The delayed reactions stress your adrenals greatly and lead to the production of cortisol as an emergency measure. The constant production of cortisol by the adrenal glands puts a strain on them, which affects their functioning.

Eat Foods That Support Adrenal Function

Now that you are taking a step towards recovery, you should get rid of programs that require you to skip meals like intermittent fasting. This makes it hard for your body to monitor your glucose levels and the amount of salt in your blood. This means you will have to obtain those nutrients through food. You can do this by consuming vegetables, quality protein, healthy fats, and carbohydrates that come from fresh fruits and starchy vegetables. Below are 'super foods' that you should definitely eat if you want to support your adrenal glands:

Proteins

Proteins help to keep your energy levels up and they do not cause spikes in your blood sugar. You should consume quality sources of proteins like free range chicken, eggs, wild fish, beef, and quality protein powder. You should always try to buy meat that is organic because it does not contain chemicals. You can purchase these at your local farmer's market.

Fats

The consumption of healthy fats is very important when

you are fighting adrenal fatigue. The secret weapon that fat has is its energy. Fats provide your body with energy that rejuvenates your adrenals and promotes their proper functioning. The best fats to consume are fats that come from natural sources. A good example of fats that you should consume includes avocado, nuts, seeds, butter, coconut, cheese, and other dairy products.

Salt

Those salt cravings that you normally get is due to low levels of aldosterone, which is a steroid hormone. It helps your body regulate its blood pressure by maintaining salt and water levels. Just like cortisol, aldosterone fluctuates during the day and is influenced by stress. Low levels of aldosterone affect your electrolyte balance. If you want to have healthy adrenals, give in to your salt cravings. Sometimes, your body knows best!

Stay Hydrated

You have probably heard how drinking water and staying hydrated is important for your health. If you are suffering from adrenal fatigue, this statement is twice as important for you. Following the 8 glasses of water per day rule is a wonderful way for you to look after your adrenal glands.

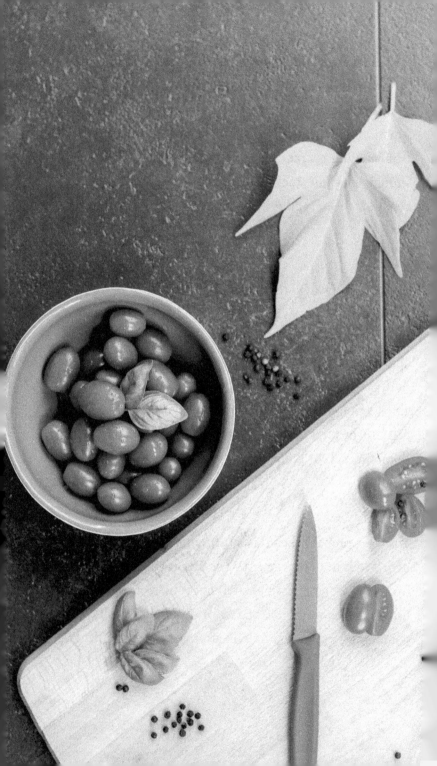

You are what you eat. This phrase could not be true enough when it comes to suffering from adrenal fatigue. Without proper nutrition, the body cannot perform as designed. Today's convenience for food has left our bodies starving for real nutrition, but what we mostly get are preservatives and chemical fillers.

Food can be broken down into three main categories. Proteins supply the body with amino acids and are responsible for aiding in the functions of the body. Fats are necessary for the body to operate but need to be consumed in healthy and moderate proportions. Carbohydrates are also an important group when it comes to adrenal function.

Carbohydrates can be classified into two categories. Sugar based carbohydrates include fructose and glucose. Starchy carbohydrates consist of vegetables, rice, and bread. When carbohydrates of any type are consumed, the body turns them into glucose. The bloodstream instantly absorbs this product and the pancreas is responsible for releasing insulin to convert the sugar in your bloodstream to energy for your body.

Since cortisol plays such a significant role in keeping the

blood sugar levels stable, the body will need to release more cortisol to keep up with a diet that is full of sugary foods. So, if you eat a cupcake late at night, this will throw off your cortisol production for the day, causing adrenal fatigue symptoms. If this is a constant routine, you will develop Adrenal Fatigue Syndrome.

Carbohydrate cycling is a term that is very popular when treating adrenal fatigue. By monitoring the amount of carbohydrates entering your body at various times of the day, you will gain instant control on the amount of glucose and insulin in your body. In return, this will help you control the cortisol levels in your body. This results in the adrenal glands being able to secrete an achievable amount of hormones within a normal time frame, instead of being constantly overworked or not able to meet the body's requirements.

The basic recipe for success when eating to cure adrenal fatigue is as follows: Three meals a day should be consumed, consisting of 1 serving of protein, 1 serving of healthy fat, and the time sensitive amount of servings of carbohydrates. Breakfast should have 1 serving; lunch should have 2 servings, and dinner should have 3 servings.

The consistent increase of carbohydrates will keep the levels of cortisol and insulin in the body at the desired amounts. Breakfast should be eaten within one hour of waking up, lunch should be eaten at about noon, and dinner should be scheduled for around 6 in the evening. Snacks are permitted since you should avoid waiting to eat until you are extremely hungry. This helps you to avoid overeating during your main meals. These snacks should be chosen by staying within the adrenal fatigue diet guidelines.

Fructose and certain proteins should be avoided at all costs. You may notice that some of these ingredients are included in the recipes in this book. These ingredients should only be used when it is absolutely necessary and only in extreme moderation. Keep this mentality when coming up with your own recipes and adrenal fatigue diet meals.

This includes:

- *brown sugar*
- *cane sugar*
- *fruit juice from concentrate*
- *granulated sugar*
- *high fructose corn syrup*
- *maple syrup*
- *molasses*
- *biscuits*
- *waffles*
- *pancakes*
- *butter*
- *milk*
- *sour cream*
- *yogurt*
- *ice cream*
- *pasta*
- *pizza crust*
- *bread*

Although this is a small list, you can see the common trend. Avoid sugary and processed foods, bulky grain-based foods, and dairy. The immediate reaction to this list is that it would be incredibly difficult to abide by.

Meal suggestions will be provided but keep in mind that it is perfectly acceptable to allow yourself a day of indulgence every now and then. If you are attempting to lose weight during the process, try to limit your indulgence day to once every 2 weeks. If you are maintaining a healthy weight, it is okay to indulge yourself once a week.

We can see that we have been eating incorrectly our whole lives. A typical breakfast can consist of eggs, pancakes, cereals, juice, and milk. This immediately sets the body and adrenal glands up for failure. The glands will go into cortisol-production overload to adjust to the levels of sugars being put into the body. Since cortisol levels are highest in the morning, breakfast is a required meal. This will help set up the metabolism and energy levels for the rest of the day.

Here is a list of foods that you should focus on and try to incorporate into your daily meals. These carbohydrates are great for the body as they originate from vegetables, fruits, and beans. Consume these foods to as it can help curb tempting carbohydrates that are full of unhealthy sugar.

- acorn squash
- barley
- beets
- black beans
- blackberries
- blueberries
- corn
- great northern beans
- kidney beans
- navy beans
- peas
- potatoes
- strawberries
- sweet potatoes

If you are on a weight loss plan as well, avoid bananas, plums, kiwi, pineapple, and watermelon until your ideal weight has been achieved.

Snacking is permitted as often as you find necessary. Ideally, when you are feeding your body the appropriate foods in the correct amounts, snacking will be limited. However, there is an extensive list of foods that can be eaten as snacks without limit.

- Asparagus
- Broccoli
- Cabbage
- Carrots
- Cauliflower
- Celery
- Cucumbers
- Garlic
- green beans
- kale
- lettuce (all forms)
- mushrooms
- onions
- peppers (all forms)
- tomatoes

Another great option when trying to consume healthier carbohydrates is to embrace juices. It allows you to have a delicious treat while still getting the nutrition from several fruits and vegetables. Certain juices can substitute a meal but be sure that you are still getting the recommended servings of protein, fat, and carbohydrates from each glass. This can be done by using protein powders or other supplements. Below, you'll find the recipes.

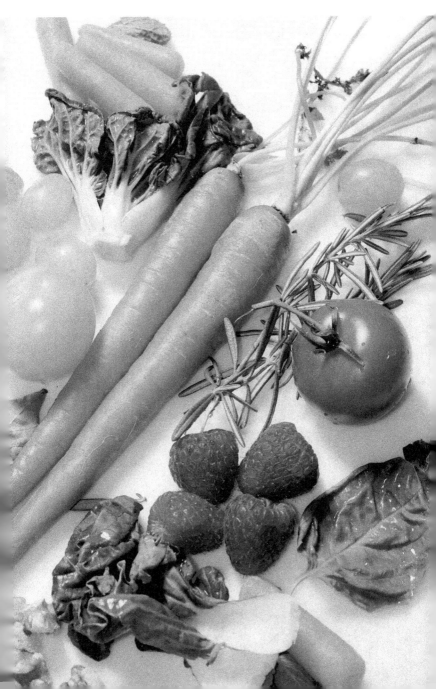

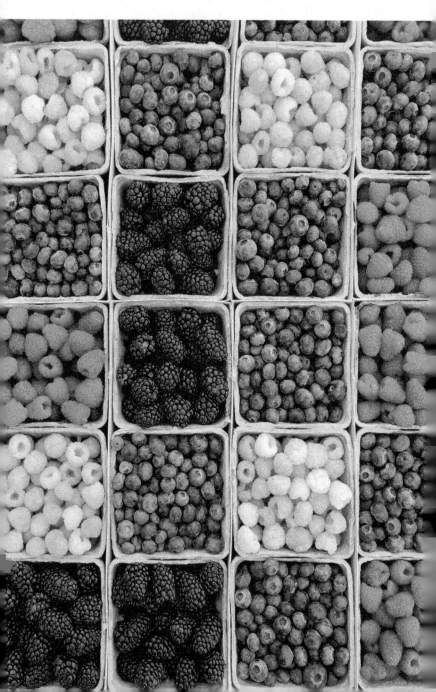

Blueberry Muffins

Serves: 2 | Prep Time: ~15 min |

Ingredients:

- 2 cups oat flour
- 2 tsp baking powder
- 1 tsp salt
- 2 eggs
- 1 lemon (grated rind and juice)
- 2 tsp vanilla
- ½ cup natural honey
- ¾ cup rice milk
- ½ tsp ground mace *nutmeg*
- 2 cups washed and dried blueberries

Total number of ingredients: 10

Eggs will provide a full amino acid profile, including tryptophan, which is a precursor to serotonin and the hormone melatonin. Blueberries will improve fatigue symptoms with their vitamin C and antioxidants.

Preparation:

1. Preheat oven to 350 degrees F.
2. Line a muffin tray with non-stick liners.

3. Mix flour, baking soda, salt, lemon rind and ground mace, eliminating all lumps.

4. Make a well in the mixture and add eggs. Beat slightly and then add lemon juice, vanilla and honey into the eggs, avoiding powder ingredients as much as possible.

5. Slowly add milk, beating lightly with a fork. Slowly incorporate the wet and dry ingredients, then gently stir in the blueberries.

6. Divide evenly into muffin liners, filling them almost to the top.

7. Bake for 25-30 minutes.

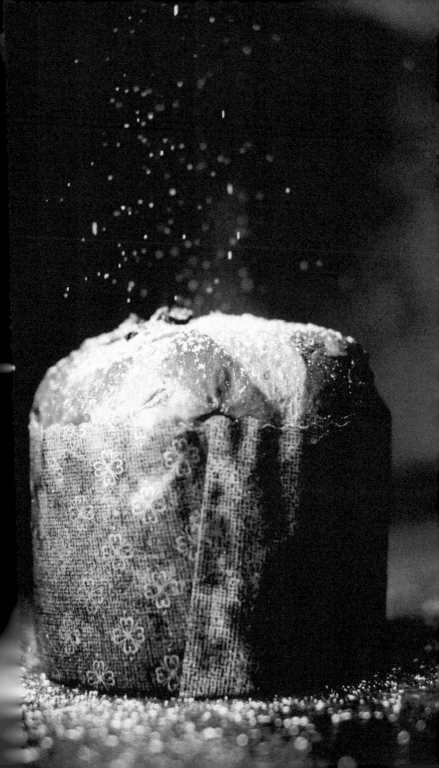

Breakfast Rice Bowl

Serves: 2 | Prep Time: ~10 min |

Ingredients:

- 1 cup rice, preferably brown
- 1 tsp honey
- ½ tsp cinnamon
- 1 apple, sliced
- Total number of ingredients: 4

White rice contains folates (vitamin B9) that will help you to not feel tired by regulating the creation of large red blood cells.

Preparation:

1. Combine all ingredients.
2. Warm in the microwave if you prefer.

Breakfast Soup

Serves: 4 | Prep Time: ~15 min |

Ingredients:

- 4 medium zucchini, sliced
- 1 pound string beans, ends removed
- 2 sticks chopped celery
- 1-2 bunches of parsley, stems removed
- 1 quart filtered water
- sea salt
- fresh herbs
- fresh whey
- Total number of ingredients: 8

Parsley contains many vitamins and minerals, including iron, vitamins C and K that will help you to manage fatigue, optimize blood clotting and avoid anemia.

Preparation:

1. Bring water to a boil and add zucchini, string beans and celery.
2. Remove from heat and add parsley.
3. Put into a blender (allow to cool slightly first) or use an immersion blender until soup has reached desired consistency.

4. Add a tsp of whey to each cup of soup before serving and season with a pinch of sea salt.

Breakfast Chili

Serves: 5 | Prep Time: ~20 min |

Ingredients:

- 1 pound lean ground turkey
- 2 tsp macadamia oil
- 1 cup mild salsa
- 1 tbsp chili powder
- 1 can black beans
- 2 cups lettuce greens
- veggies and garnishes (onions, mushrooms, parsley)

Total number of ingredients: 9

Black beans contain important minerals and antioxidants, such as manganese and magnesium, that help with release of neurotransmitters like serotonin and dopamine.

Preparation:

1. Brown the ground turkey in the oil.
2. Add salsa, beans, greens and chili powder.
3. Add any other desired veggies and cook until tender.
4. Garnish as desired.

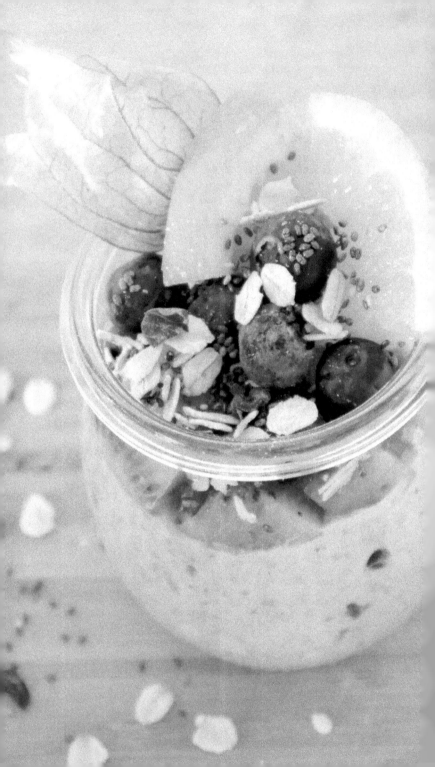

FRUIT PORRIDGE

Serves: 1 | Prep Time: ~15 min |

Ingredients:

- ½ cup rolled oats
- ½ cup nut milk
- dash of cinnamon
- ¼ tsp pure vanilla
- 1 kiwi
- ¼ cup strawberries
- ¼ cup coconut flakes
- ¼ cup cashews
- Total number of ingredients: 8

Oats contain zinc which plays a role in testosterone production; hence, it improves neurotransmitter production. Kiwi is a great source of vitamin C, which is important for serotonin production and fatigue management

Preparation:

1. Put the oats, milk and cinnamon into a glass jar and place in the refrigerator overnight.
2. In the morning, bake cashews and coconut flakes in the oven for 7 minutes 300F or 150C.
3. Place cashews, coconut and fruit on top of the oats.

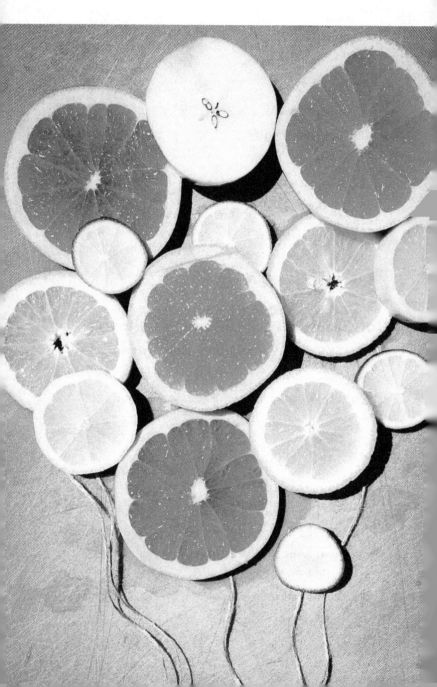

BROCCOLI SALAD

Serves: 2 | Prep Time: ~15 min |

Ingredients:

- 1 tbsp whole grain mustard
- 1 tbsp sherry vinegar
- 3 tbsp extra virgin olive oil
- 1 head broccoli
- 1 avocado
- handful roasted almonds

Total number of ingredients: 6

Chronic olive oil consumption is associated with an increase in dopamine, norepinephrine, GABA and serotonin levels.

Preparation:

1. Combine mustard, vinegar and olive oil.
2. Chop broccoli and add to the dressing.
3. Cut and slice avocado. Add to the dressing.
4. Shake to cover evenly and top with almonds.

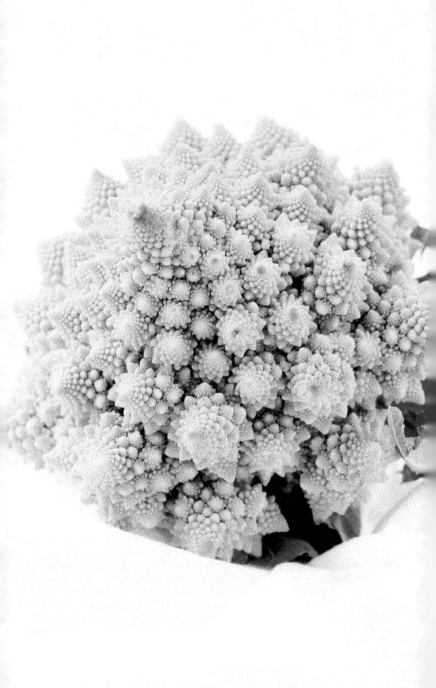

Beet and Sweet Potato Berry Salad

Serves: 3 | Prep Time: ~15 min |

Ingredients:

- 1 sweet potato
- ¼ cup mixed, dried fruits (cranberries, strawberries, raspberries, and/or blackberries)
- 4 beets (peeled)
- ¼ cup pecans (chopped)
- 1 bunch of kale (chopped and blanched)
- salt and pepper to taste
- 1 tbsp olive oil

Dressing:

- 2 tbsp apple cider vinegar
- lemon juice to taste
- 1 tsp wasabi
- ¼ cup olive oil

Total number of ingredients: 15

Pecans contain thiamine (vitamin B1), which plays role in the production of neurotransmitter acetylcholine.

Directions:

1. Preheat the oven to 350 F.
2. Dice the sweet potato and beets into cubes and place on baking sheet with salt, pepper, and a drizzle of olive oil. Bake for 30-45 minutes and toss intermittently until potatoes and beets are soft.
3. Add the potatoes, beets, kale, dried fruits, and pecans to a bowl and toss.
4. Blend dressing ingredients and add atop the other ingredients in the bowl, then toss the salad again.

FRUIT-STUFFED ACORN SQUASH

Serves: 4 | Prep Time: ~15 min |

Ingredients:

- 2 medium acorn squash (cut in half and pitted)
- ¼ tsp each: salt, cinnamon, nutmeg
- ¾ cup blackberries, raspberries, and cranberries
- 2 cups apples (chopped)
- ¼ cup coconut sugar
- 2 tbsp coconut oil

Total number of ingredients: 10

A recipe with healthy ingredients: healthy fats, starchy carbs and a decent amount of protein. Coconut oil contains saturated fatty acids that increase cholesterol, testosterone and, hence, neurotransmitter release.

Directions:

1. Place squash, with the inside facing down, on a non-greased baking tray and bake at about 300 F for 20 minutes.
2. Mix the rest of the ingredients aside from the salt.
3. Remove from the oven and flip squash over. Sprinkle on the salt and spoon in the mix.
4. Bake for another 45 minutes or until tender.

BARLEY FRUIT BREAD

Serves: 10 slices | Prep Time: ~10 min |

Ingredients:

- 3 cups barley flour
- 1 tsp salt
- 2 ½ tbsp baking powder
- 2 tbsp of honey
- ¼ cup canola oil
- 2 eggs
- 1 cup almond milk
- ½ cup of dried blackberries, strawberries, and raspberries

Total number of ingredients: 10

Barley flour and healthy fruits are great foods that will help prevent adrenal dysfunction.

Directions:

1. Preheat oven to 350 F.
2. Mix the dry ingredients in one bowl, and the wet ingredients in another.
3. Once each mixture is well combined, add them together.
4. Pour the mixture in a greased loaf pan.
5. Bake for 20-30 minutes.

Bean Berry Mexican Salad with Avocado Dressing

Serves: 4 | Prep Time: ~15 min |

Ingredients:

Salad:

- 1 cup mixed berries (blueberries, raspberries, and blackberries)
- 2 eight-ounce cans of black beans
- 1 cup cherry tomatoes (halved)
- 1 cup corn
- 2 cups baby romaine
- 1 cup of cilantro (chopped)

Avocado dressing:

- ¼ cup lime (about 3 limes)
- 1 avocado
- salt and pepper according to taste
- 1 cup fresh cilantro (chopped)
- 3 tbsp olive oil
- 1 jalapeño (if you aren't a spice lover, only use about half)

Total number of ingredients: 15

This recipe comes with starchy carbohydrates that will help your body and its adrenal glands function well. Berries contain many antioxidants that will improve neurotransmitter release.

Directions:

1. For the dressing, blend all the ingredients in a blender until smooth.
2. For the salad, add the lettuce, tomato, corn, beans, berries, and cilantro in a large salad bowl.
3. Add the dressing on top and toss well.

VEGGIE PLATE

Serves: 1 | Prep Time: ~10 min |

Ingredients:

- 1 tomato, sliced
- 1 bell pepper, sliced
- ½ cucumber, sliced
- ½ cup broccoli
- 1 cup Greek yogurt
- salmon, chicken, turkey, or hard-boiled eggs for protein

Total number of ingredients: 6

Tomato and other veggies are rich in fiber that will decrease blood glucose spikes and improve your fatigue.

Preparation:

1. Arrange veggies on a plate with yogurt for dipping.
2. Serve with protein source of choice.

Breadless Sandwich

Serves: 1 | Prep Time: ~15 min |

Ingredients:

- 1 large lettuce leaf
- ¼ cup organic hummus
- tomato slices
- cucumber slices
- spinach leaves
- ½ cup tuna
- Total number of ingredients: 6

Tuna contains omega-3 fatty acids that will improve your brain function.

Preparation:

1. Place all ingredients on a lettuce leaf in the same way you would construct a sandwich.
2. Enjoy!

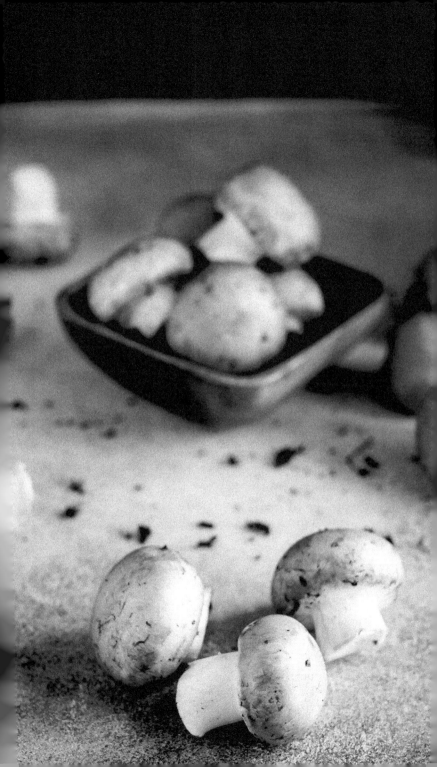

MUSHROOM MUFFINS

Serves: 2 | Prep Time: ~15 min |

Ingredients:

- 4 tsp macadamia oil
- 2 cups sliced button mushrooms
- 1 red bell pepper, diced
- 1 small red onion, diced
- 2 garlic cloves, minced
- ½ tsp sea salt
- ½ tsp freshly ground black pepper
- ½ tsp chili powder
- ½ tsp ground turmeric
- 1 cup canned green lentils, rinsed
- 1 cup diced cooked chicken breast
- ½ cup garbanzo bean flour

Total number of ingredients: 12

Lentils are a great source of protein, iron, complex carbs and fiber that will improve your fatigue through different mechanisms.

Preparation:

1. Preheat the oven to 350 degrees F.
2. Line a muffin tray with non-stick muffin liners.

3. Sauté the mushrooms, red pepper, and onion over low heat in the macadamia oil.
4. Add the garlic and other seasonings.
5. Stir well and add the lentils and chicken.
6. Once mixed, add the flour and blend. Gently incorporate, taking care not to over-mix.
7. Evenly distribute between muffin liners and bake for 20 to 25 minutes.

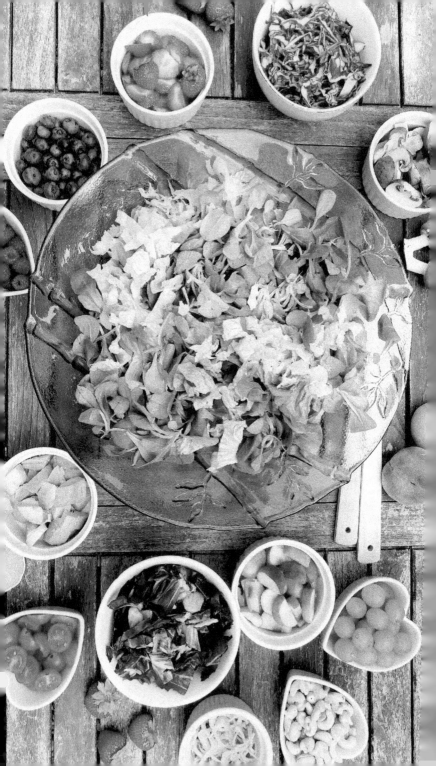

Raspberry and Spinach Salad

Serves: 2 | Prep Time: ~15 min |

Ingredients:

- 3 tbsp olive oil
- 2 tbsp raspberry vinegar
- ¼ cup fresh raspberries, pureed
- 8 cups baby spinach
- 2 cups fresh raspberries
- 4 tbsp crushed walnuts
- ½ of a red onion, chopped
- 3 kiwis, peeled and sliced
- sea salt and black pepper to taste

Total number of ingredients: 10

The majority of these ingredients will provide you with a ton of micronutrients (like iron, vitamin C, E, etc.) for increased neurotransmitter release and better fatigue management.

Directions:

1. Combine olive oil, vinegar and pureed raspberries and mix to make the dressing.
2. In a separate bowl, combine spinach, raspberries, walnuts, kiwis and onion.
3. Drizzle with the dressing and toss to coat.
4. Serve immediately.

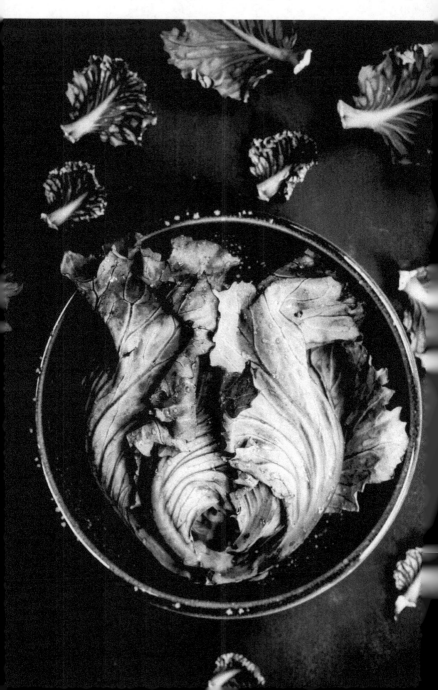

Beef Stir Fry

Serves: 2 | Prep Time: ~15 min |

Ingredients:

- 1 tsp toasted sesame oil
- 1 pound boneless beef steak, thinly sliced
- 2 pounds bok choy, sliced and separated
- 2 garlic cloves, minced
- 2 pinches freshly ground black pepper
- 1 pinch sea salt
- Total number of ingredients: 6

Beef is a good source of protein, iron and zinc, which all play a role in testosterone production and decreased adrenal fatigue.

Directions:

1. Heat the sesame oil and cook the steak until browned, about 3 minutes.
2. Add the bok choy stems and garlic and sauté until browned, about 1 minute.
3. Add bok choy leaves and cook for at least 5 minutes.
4. Season with pepper and salt to taste.
5. Serve hot with a small portion of rice.

FISH, BEANS, VEGGIES & SWEET POTATO DISH

Serves: 4 | Prep Time: ~15 min |

Ingredients:

- 4 medium sweet potatoes
- 2 cups brown rice
- 3 tbsp olive oil
- 3 tbsp freshly chopped parsley and basil
- 4 six-ounce tilapia fillets
- salt, pepper, and paprika to desired taste
- 1 eight-oz. can black beans
- 3 cups mixed chopped veggies
  (carrots, peas, corn, green beans)

Total number of ingredients: 13

Great recipe for healthy fuel, low GI foods with good protein and lots of veggies! Brown rice contains a lot of vitamins, including vitamin B6 and thiamine (vitamin B1) that will increase your serotonin levels.

Directions:

1. Preheat oven to 350 F.
2. Cook the rice as instructed on the packet. Once done, cover till later.

3. Rub the fillet with olive oil, parsley, basil, salt, pepper, and paprika and place on a lightly oiled oven tray.

4. With the skin still on, roughly chop the potatoes into wedge shapes. Top with pepper, salt, and chili powder (optional), place on the same oiled tray as the tilapia, and place in the preheated oven.

5. While the wedges and fish are cooking, place the veggies in a lightly oiled pan and let cook till soft.

6. Take the oven tray out when fish is suitably cooked (probably 20-30 minutes).

7. On a plate, add a piece of tilapia, a handful of wedges, a proportional amount of rice and beans, and some of the vegetables. Add additional spices as desired.

Chicken-Bean Stir-fry

Serves: 4 | Prep Time: ~20 min |

Ingredients:

- 1 large onion (chopped)
- 1 tbsp red pepper flakes
- 3 tbsp olive oil
- 4 cloves of garlic (minced)
- 4 boneless chicken breasts (cut into strips)
- 2 tsp cumin
- 2 tsp oregano
- 2 cans of black beans
- 3 tbsp balsamic vinegar
- 3 cups chicken broth
- 1 ½ cups white rice
- salt and pepper to taste

Total number of ingredients: 13

A list of various ingredients that will help you enjoy a healthy dinner meal. Chicken will help boost your norepinephrine and serotonin levels.

Directions:

1. In an oiled pan, add the pepper flakes, garlic, and onion and cook until tender.

2. Increase the heat and add the chicken until it cooks through.
3. Lower the heat and add the cumin and oregano and let simmer for 1 minute. Add in the beans, remaining spices, and vinegar. Mix well and let simmer for 30 minutes.
4. In another pan, add broth and rice and cook for 20 minutes until rice is cooked.
5. Pour the chicken and bean mixture over the rice and mix well.
6. Serve.

CORN AND BEAN-FILLED POTATOES

Serves: 8 | Prep Time: ~15 min |

Ingredients:

- 4 large potatoes
- ½ cups onion (diced)
- 1 tsp cumin
- 2 tsp garlic (minced)
- ½ tsp chili powder
- 2 cups black beans (drained)
- 1 cup frozen corn
- 1 cup salsa
- ¼ cup fresh cilantro (chopped)
- ¼ cup shredded cheddar cheese (optional)

Total number of ingredients: 10

This recipe will fuel your body with complex, healthy carbohydrates that are a great source of energy because they don't produce insulin spikes and release energy in a more efficient way.

Directions:

1. Cut the potatoes in half long ways and scoop them out until only the intact skin is left.
2. Mash the scooped out potato in a bowl and add in

cumin, onions, cilantro, chili powder, black beans, garlic, and corn and mix.

3. Spoon the mixture back into the empty potato skins and add the salsa and cheese (if desired) on top.

4. Bake for about 15-20 minutes at 400 F or until the cheese appears to have melted.

Veggie Pot Pie

Serves: 5 | Prep Time: ~20 min |

Ingredients:

- ½ medium onion (chopped)
- 2 cups veggie broth
- 1 clove of garlic (minced)
- 2 cups mixed frozen veggies (carrots, corn, peas, and beets)
- ¼ cup almond milk
- ¼ cup almond flour
- 2 bay leaves
- salt and pepper (added to taste)
- puff pastry or pie crust of choice

Like the previous recipe, the Veggie Pot Pie will fuel your body with complex, starchy carbohydrates.

Directions:

1. Preheat the oven to 425 F.
2. Add the onion and garlic into a lightly oiled pan and cook for about 5 minutes until soft.
3. Add the almond flour then whisk.
4. Add and stir in the veggie broth.
5. Add almond milk and bay leaves and stir some more. Let simmer until mixture has thickened (about 10 minutes). Note: (if the mixture is not thickening, scoop out

a ½ cup of broth and add two more tablespoons of almond flour).

6. Add the veggies and allow it to cook for 5 more minutes.

7. Taste the mixture and add seasoning as desired.

8. Remove bay leaves and add the mixture into an 8x8 inch baking dish.

9. Top the mixture with your uncooked homemade or store-bought biscuits.

10. Keep in the oven for about 20-30 minutes before serving.

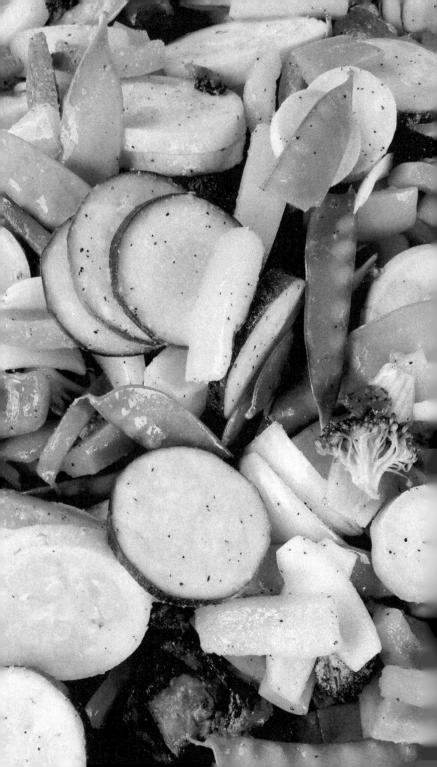

Veggie Soup with Beans and Potatoes

Serves: 8 | Prep Time: ~15 min |

Ingredients:

- 1 large onion (chopped)
- 1 tbsp olive oil
- 3 large garlic cloves (minced)
- 1 chopped carrot (diced)
- ½ cup peas
- 2 medium sized potatoes (cubed with the skin)
- 1 cup mushrooms (chopped)
- 1 ½ cups black beans (canned and drained)
- 1 ½ cups red kidney beans (canned and brained)
- 8 cups of water
- pinch of salt, pepper, cumin, and chili powder (add until you reach your desired preference)
- 1 bay leaf
- 1 sprig of rosemary
- ¾ cup spinach
- 1 tsp vinegar

Total number of ingredients: 17

> *And again, beans are a great source of protein, complex carbs, fiber and magnesium, which helps to normalize neurotransmitters and stress hormones.*

Directions:

1. Throw onions, garlic, bay leaf, and rosemary sprig into an oiled soup pot on medium heat and cook until onions are soft (be careful as you will have to spoon out the bay leaf and rosemary later).
2. Add the potatoes, peas, and carrots and cook for about 5 minutes. Then add in the water.
3. Add in the mushrooms and beans and allow the mixture to come to a boil.
4. Allow it to simmer for about 20 minutes and then spoon out the bay leaf and rosemary sprig if you can (if not, just expect it to pop up when you are eating!).
5. Add in the spinach and spices as desired and allow it to cook for another 10 minutes.

CABBAGE ROLL CASSEROLE

Serves: 8 | Prep Time: ~15 min |

Ingredients:

- 1 small head green cabbage, chopped
- 1 pound of lean ground turkey
- 1 small onion, chopped
- minced garlic to taste
- ½ head of cauliflower, diced
- 3 cans tomato sauce
- 2 tbsp lemon juice
- 2 tbsp honey
- sea salt and pepper to taste

Total number of ingredients: 10

Besides being a great source of protein, turkey contains selenium which provides a faster neurotransmitter release.

Directions:

1. Preheat the oven to 350 F.
2. Prepare a 9x13 inch pan and brown the turkey.
3. Add onions and cook until tender.
4. Add cauliflower and simmer until soft.
5. Add tomato sauce, lemon juice, honey, garlic, salt and pepper.

6. Continue simmering, stirring occasionally, for about 10 minutes.
7. Place cabbage in the bottom of the pan.
8. Cover with the meat mixture.
9. Spread evenly and place in the oven for about 30 minutes, or until bubbly.

Meatloaf

Serves: 6 | Prep Time: ~20 min |

Ingredients:

- 1-pound lean ground turkey
- 2 eggs
- 2 cups tomato sauce, divided
- 5 cloves garlic, minced
- 1 poblano pepper
- 1 cup baby spinach, chopped
- 1 tsp rosemary, chopped
- 1 tsp basil, chopped
- 1 tsp oregano, chopped
- sea salt and pepper to taste

Total number of ingredients: 10

Eggs provide the amino acid tryptophan which will increase your serotonin levels.

Directions:

1. Preheat oven to 400 degrees F.
2. Combine all ingredients (except for 1 cup of tomato sauce) together in a bowl and place in the refrigerator for about an hour.
3. Prepare a loaf pan. Shape meat mixture and place in pan.

4. Top with tomato sauce.
5. Bake for 75 minutes or until browned and cooked thoroughly.

Multi-Bean Chili

Serves: 6 | Prep Time: ~20 min |

Ingredients:

- 1 onion (diced)
- 1 tbsp canola oil
- 3 tbsp chili powder
- 4 garlic cloves (minced)
- 1 tbsp cumin
- ½ tsp cayenne pepper
- 3 cups crushed tomatoes
- 2 cups black beans (canned)
- 2 cups red kidney beans (canned)
- 2 cups navy beans (canned)
- 3 small tomatoes (chopped)
- 3 cups water
- salt and pepper added to taste
- Total number of ingredients: 14

Tomatoes contain vitamin C and choline which will improve your acetylcholine levels and help decrease fatigue.

Directions:

1. In a pot, add the canola oil and onions and cook until soft.

2. Add in chili powder, garlic, cumin, and cayenne pepper and cook for about 1 minute.
3. Stir in the beans, canned and fresh tomatoes, water, and salt and pepper to taste and bring to a boil.
4. Allow it to simmer 15 more minutes until done.

CHICKEN LETTUCE WRAPS

Serves: 6 | Prep Time: ~15 min |

Ingredients:

- 2 tbsp coconut oil
- 1 inch piece of fresh ginger, diced
- 3 garlic cloves, diced
- 3 chicken breasts, cut into cubes
- ½ tsp crushed red pepper
- 1 green pepper, diced
- ½ cup button mushrooms, diced
- 4 green onions, sliced
- 2 tbsp gluten-free tamari
- sea salt and pepper to taste
- 1 head of bibb lettuce, rinsed, separated, and dried

Total number of ingredients: 12

Chicken breasts will provide a lot of glutamic acid which will increase neurotransmitter glutamate levels.

Directions:

1. Sauté ginger and garlic in the coconut oil.
2. Add chicken and crushed red pepper and cook for 5-7 minutes or until cooked through.

3. Add bell pepper and mushrooms and cook until tender.
4. Add the scallion with the tamari.
5. Season to taste and serve in lettuce leaves.

BUTTERNUT SQUASH AND KALE CURRY

Serves: 4 | Prep Time: ~20 min |

Ingredients:

- 1 onion, chopped
- 1 butternut squash, chopped into small cubes
- 1 bunch kale, chopped
- 1 can chickpeas
- 1 can coconut milk
- 2 tbsp yellow curry paste
- 1 ½ cups vegetable stock
- 2 tbsp fish sauce
- 1 tbsp brown sugar
- 1 lime
- ¼ bunch cilantro, chopped

Total number of ingredients: 11

Chickpeas contain the amino acid Phenylalanine which is eventually converted to dopamine, noradrenaline and adrenaline.

Directions:

1. Whisk curry paste into half the can of coconut milk in a saucepan.
2. Add onion and simmer.

3. Add squash, kale and chickpeas along with the rest of the coconut milk.
4. Add vegetable stock, fish sauce and brown sugar.
5. Keep pan covered and bring to a boil.
6. Lower heat and let simmer for 10 minutes.
7. Add kale and continue simmering for a few more minutes.
8. Add juice from half of the lime, more fish sauce, and brown sugar or lime juice to taste.

BEAN VEGGIE BOWL

Serves: 1 | Prep Time: ~15 min |

Ingredients:

- 1 cup frozen veggies (green beans, carrots, broccoli, and corn)
- 1 can kidney beans
- ½ cup onion (chopped)
- ½ cup celery (chopped)
- ½ cup green pepper (chopped)
- salt and pepper
- 5 medium-sized lettuce pieces
- lemon juice

Total number of ingredients: 12

A good mix of veggies that contain a lot of antioxidants which protect the nitrergic neurotransmitters.

Directions:

1. Cook the frozen veggies until thawed and mix in the beans.
2. Transfer to a bowl, and add the onion, celery, and green pepper.
3. Mix together and add lemon juice, salt, and pepper to taste.
4. Spoon onto good-sized lettuce pieces and serve.

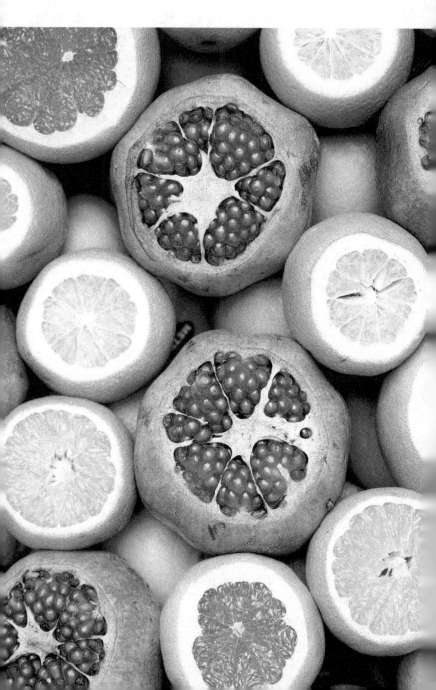

Coconut Honey Bites

Serves: 6 | Prep Time: ~10 min |

Ingredients:

- 1 cup solid coconut oil
- 2 tbsp honey

Total number of ingredients: 2

Coconut oil is rich in saturated fats that increase your testosterone and neurotransmitter release.

Directions:

1. Combine and blend in a blender. They must fully incorporate.
2. Place in molds or in a shallow glass pan and freeze.
3. Cut into squares or remove from mold when ready to consume.

GELATIN TREATS

Serves: 4 | Prep Time: ~10 min |

Ingredients:

- 1 pound organic strawberries, tops removed
- 2 cups very hot water
- 3 tulsi tea bags
- 4 tbsp grass-fed gelatin
- ¾ tsp liquid stevia

Total number of ingredients: 5

Strawberries are a source of vitamin C and choline, which increase acetylcholine levels and decrease fatigue.

Directions:

1. Pour the hot water into a bowl and allow the tea bags to soak for 10 minutes.
2. Blend the strawberries in a blender until smooth.
3. Add the tea, gelatin and stevia to the strawberries.
4. Whisk to combine and pour into a glass pan.
5. Refrigerate until gelatin has set. Cut into squares.

CABBAGE KALE SALAD

Serves: 2 | Prep Time: ~15 min |

Ingredients:

- 5 cups green cabbage (chopped)
- ½ cup walnuts (chopped)
- ½ cup feta cheese
- ½ red pepper (shredded)
- ½ cup carrots (shredded)
- 1 lemon's juice
- 2 tbsp olive oil
- salt and pepper
- 3 cups kale (chopped)

Total number of ingredients: 9

Healthy ingredients to consume as a snack; mix it up in a salad and enjoy! Kale is a good source of organic sulphur which will boost your GABA levels.

Directions:

1. In a bowl, combine the cheese, walnuts, cabbage, kale, carrots, and peppers.
2. In another bowl, mix the oil, salt, pepper, and lemon juice.
3. Pour the dressing mixture over the salad and toss.

Veggies and Hummus

Serves: 5 | Prep Time: ~20 min |

Ingredients:

- vegetables as desired (cucumber, pepper, tomato)
- 7 ounces canned chickpeas
- 2 cloves garlic
- 1 tbsp Greek yogurt
- 1 tbsp sesame oil
- 2 tbsp olive oil
- 3 tbsp lemon juice
- 1 pinch sugar
- 1 tsp chili powder
- 1 tsp paprika
- 2 tbsp finely chopped parsley
- sea salt and pepper to taste

Total number of ingredients: 15

Directions:

1. Combine all ingredients (except vegetables) in a blender and combine thoroughly.
2. Dip vegetables in hummus.

Simple Avocado-Veggie Salad

Serves: 1 | Prep Time: ~15 min |

Ingredients:

Salad:

- ¼ cup avocado (diced)
- ¼ cup mushrooms (chopped)
- ¼ cup cauliflower (florets)
- ¼ cup broccoli (floret)
- ¼ cup carrots (shredded)

Dressing:

- 1 tbsp Dijon mustard
- salt and pepper
- lemon juice to taste

Total number of ingredients: 10

Another salad with ingredients to consume without limits. Cauliflower and broccoli contain a lot of choline which will boost your acetylcholine levels.

Directions:

1. Blend all dressing ingredients and adjust to desired preference.

2. Toss other ingredients in a bowl and mix in the dressing.

Kale Rainbow Salad

Serves: 3 | Prep Time: ~20 min |

Ingredients:

Dressing:

- ½ cup lemon juice
- 2 garlic cloves (minced)
- 2 tsp olive oil
- salt and pepper

Salad:

- 6 cups kale
- ½ cup baby tomatoes
- 1 cup red pepper (diced)
- 1 cup yellow pepper (diced)
- 1 cup carrots (shredded)
- ½ cup onion (diced)
- ½ cup cilantro (chopped)
- ½ cup parsley (chopped)
- ¼ cup almonds (roasted)
- ½ avocado (chopped)

Total number of ingredients: 14

Excellent salad to consume when you start feeling hungry. It takes some time to prepare but tastes amazing! Kale provides sulphur, which is necessary for GABA production.

Directions:

1. Blend dressing ingredients and set aside.
2. Put the kale and all the vegetables, aside from the parsley, avocado, and cilantro in a bowl.
3. Add the dressing on top with the cilantro and parsley and mix.
4. Refrigerate for 20 minutes, toss again, and add the avocado and almonds.

MASHED CAULIFLOWER

Serves: 3 | Prep Time: ~15 min |

Ingredients:

- ¼ head cauliflower, cut into small bites
- sea salt and pepper to taste

Total number of ingredients: 10

> *Cauliflower contains a lot of choline which will boost your acetylcholine levels.*

Directions:

1. Place cauliflower in a saucepan and cover with water.
2. Boil until tender.
3. Drain and mash until desired consistency is achieved.
4. Season with salt and pepper as desired.

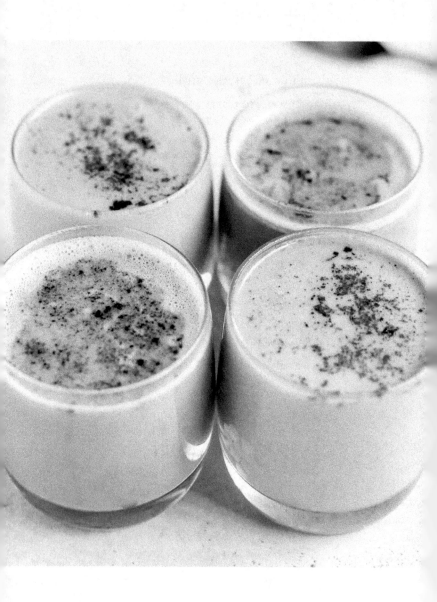

KALE SMOOTHIE

Serves: 4 | Prep Time: ~10 min |

Ingredients:

- 3 cups kale
- 1 tbsp supergreens powder
- 1 cup frozen organic blueberries
- 1 tsp maca
- 1-2 tbsp MCT oil
- 1 lemon, skin removed
- 2-4 drops stevia
- 1 cup water

Total number of ingredients: 8

Best consumed as a breakfast smoothie. Kale is a great source of organic sulfur which is a necessary component to generate GABA.

Directions:

1. Blend until completely combined.
2. Serve cold.

Avocado Smoothie

Serves: 1 | Prep Time: ~10 min |

Ingredients:

- 2 cups cold water
- 1 avocado, peeled and pitted
- ½ cup fresh parsley
- 1 apple, cored and seeded
- 1 carrot, cut into chunks
- 1 lemon, skin peeled off
- 1 kale leaf
- 1 piece of fresh ginger root
- Total number of ingredients: 8

Directions:

1. Blend until completely combined.
2. Serve.

Sweet and Sour Drink

Serves: 1 | Prep Time: ~10 min |

Ingredients:

- 2 tbsp apple cider vinegar
- 1 tbsp lime juice concentrated
- 4 tsp stevia

Total number of ingredients: 3

Directions:

1. Combine all ingredients over ice and stir.
2. Enjoy immediately.

Strawberry Banana Power Smoothie

Serves: 2 | Prep Time: ~10 min |

Ingredients:

- 1 banana
- 1 cup frozen strawberries
- 1 cup frozen blueberries
- 1 cup spinach
- 1 tbsp coconut oil
- 2 tbsp chia seeds
- 1 cup yogurt
- stevia to taste

Total number of ingredients: 8

Chia seeds are a good source of omega-3 fatty acids which increase brain function. Berries and spinach provide micronutrients for a more efficient neurotransmitter release.

Directions:

1. Blend until completely combined.
2. Serve chilled.

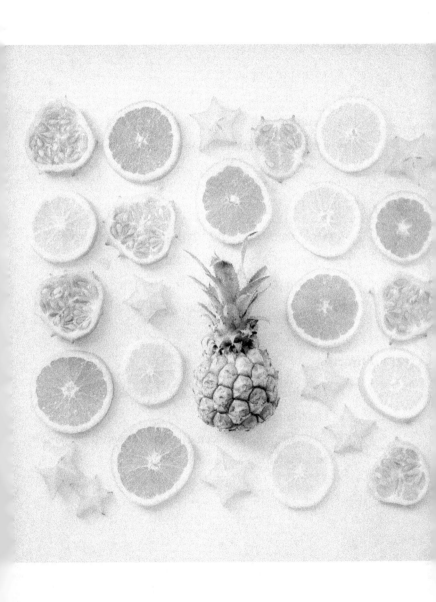

PINEAPPLE POWER JUICE

Serves: 2 | Prep Time: ~10 min |

Ingredients:

- 1 cup pineapple
- 1 cup carrots
- 1 cup spinach
- cardamom and cinnamon to taste

Total number of ingredients: 4

> *Spinach contains iron that will help decrease your fatigue levels. Pineapple is a great source of vitamin C which is necessary for serotonin production.*

Directions:

1. Combine ingredients in a blender with a juicer attachment.
2. After the juice has been extracted, top with cardamom and cinnamon as desired.

FOODS AND RECIPES TO RESTORE OR BOOST NEUROTRANSMITTER BALANCES

✓ *Turkey:*

Tryptophan is an important amino acid found in all protein foods; the highest amounts are found in turkey. This amino acid is essential for the production of serotonin and dopamine. Without enough tryptophan, your neurotransmitter levels will fall. When you eat turkey along with a small amount of carbohydrates, all of the amino acids except for tryptophan are cleared from the bloodstream, leaving tryptophan free to form both serotonin and dopamine.

✓ *Flaxseed:*

Flaxseeds contain both tryptophan and high levels of omega 3 fatty acids. More than 50% of the brain is made of structural fats, and omega 3 fatty acids make up a large proportion of brain nerve cells.

✓ *Fish or Seafood:*

Most people know different kinds of fish are good for you, but salmon, sardines, and herring are especially rich in oils containing the essential fats EPA and DHA, which have been shown to increase neurotransmitter levels.

✓ *Buckwheat:*

Buckwheat, a natural starch food, is particularly rich in many B vitamins, including vitamin B6. Research has shown that vitamin B6 is directly involved in proper serotonin synthesis in the brain. Eating buckwheat alone won't affect your serotonin or dopamine levels, but eating it along with a protein high in tryptophan will help stimulate neurotransmitter production.

✓ *Whey Protein:*

Whey has been proven to stimulate your appetite, improve insulin sensitivity, and bolster the immune system. It has also been shown to be a great protein to pair with a workout. Whey protein has also been shown to increase serotonin levels.

✓ *Bananas:*

Bananas contain tryptophan and a good amount of carbohydrates, including sugars. Bananas also contain inulin, which is prebiotic with numerous health benefits. So, you wouldn't want to eat a banana per day, but maybe one or two per week to mix things up a bit.

✓ *Eggs:*

Eggs are a source of saturated fats and cholesterol, which will increase your own cholesterol levels and be converted into testosterone. Higher testosterone levels will, in turn, raise neurotransmitter levels, as well as promote increased muscle growth and fat loss.

✓ *Sour Cherries:*

Sour cherries contain melatonin, which aids in getting a good, restful night's sleep. The body replenishes its serotonin and dopamine supply mostly during sleep.

✓ *Avocado, walnuts, asparagus, beef, spinach, dark chocolate, pineapple, oats, and pecans.*

✓ *Serotonin and dopamine levels can be increased by these foods.*

MORE BRAIN FOOD

Another way to keep those neurotransmitters flowing is to strive to have a healthy sex life. Sexual intercourse dramatically increases serotonin, dopamine, and many other essential neurotransmitters. There are many healthy foods that can help stimulate a healthy libido.

✓ *Watermelon:*

Watermelon contains high amounts of citrulline, an amino acid that helps improve blood flow to the heart and genitalia, as well as the rest of the body.

✓ *Dark Chocolate:*

Again, dark chocolate. Well, dark chocolate not only contains serotonin, which boosts your mood, it also contains phenyl ethylamine, which mimics the brain chemistry of a person in love.

✓ *Asparagus:*

Asparagus is high in folate, a B vitamin that helps increase histamine levels. Histamine plays an essential role in sex drive for both men and women.

✓ *Oysters:*

Oysters boost dopamine and are full of zinc, which is needed for testosterone production. If you don't care for oysters, you could purchase a zinc supplement instead.

✓ *Pumpkin Seeds:*

Pumpkin seeds are another great source of zinc and are also rich in omega 3 fatty acids, which act as a precursor of prostaglandins. Prostaglandins play a key role in sexual health. Important note: Zinc deficiency can make a woman completely lose her sex drive.

✓ *Garlic:*

Besides causing bad breath, garlic also contains allicin, a compound thought to increase blood flow to the sex organs.

✓ *Avocados:*

High in vitamin B6, which increases male hormone production and potassium to regulate a woman's thyroid gland, avocados can play an important role in boosting libido for both sexes. They're also rich in folic acid, which helps to increase energy and stamina.

✓ *chili's:*

Chilies are hot because they have a lot of capsaicin, a

chemical which also increases blood flow and triggers the release of mood-enhancing endorphins.

✓ *Nutmeg:*

Used for centuries in Indian medicine to boost libido, at least one animal study has shown an extract of nutmeg to have the same effect on mating behavior as Viagra.

✓ *Celery:*

Raw celery increases production of androsterone, an odourless hormone released when a man perspires. While you can't smell it, androsterone apparently acts as a pheromone, triggering female attraction.

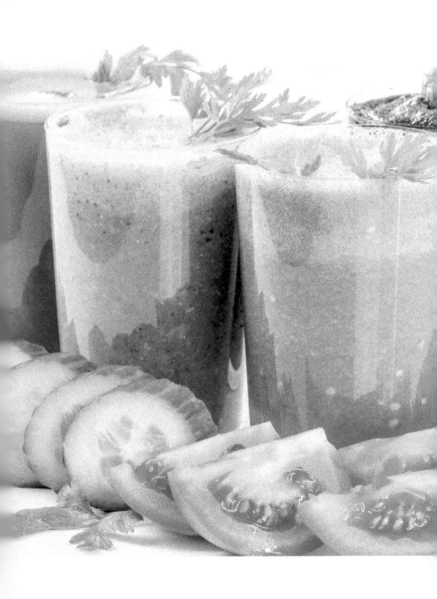

Chocolate Beet Superfood Smoothie

Serves: 2 | Prep Time: ~10 min |

Ingredients:

- 1 small beet, peeled
- ½ banana
- ½ cup mixed berries
- 1 tsp of maca
- 1 tbsp of raw cacao powder
- 1 tbsp of chia seeds
- 2 cups water
- a handful of greens (spinach for example)

Total number of ingredients: 8

Cacao helps you boost your serotonin level and contains phenyl ethylamine. Beets, berries and spinach are great sources of vitamins and minerals.

Directions:

1. Place all the above ingredients in a blender and blend thoroughly. Transfer into a glass and serve.

   - *Beets are a source of betalains phytonutrients. They provide detox support, anti-inflammatory effects, and antioxidants.*

   - *Berries are a source of antioxidants and low glycaemic.*

   - *Chia seeds: eat them to get fiber, protein, and good fats.*

   - *Raw cacao provides antioxidants and minerals like manganese, zinc, iron, copper, magnesium, potassium, and calcium.*

   - *Maca is a hormone regulator with lots of vitamin E, C and B-complex. It also nourishes the nervous system.*

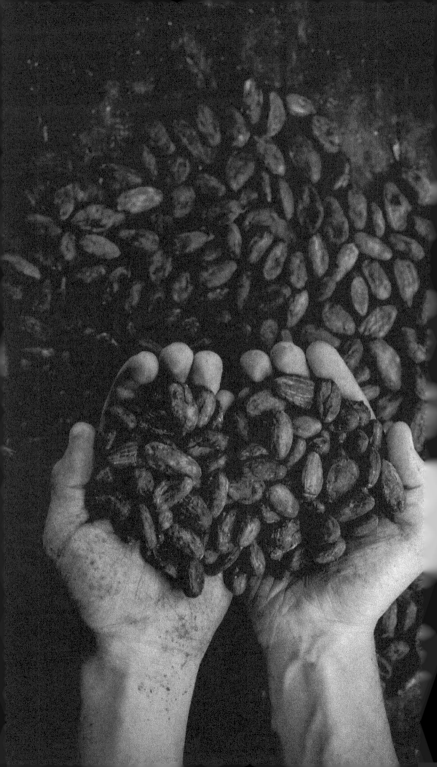

STIR FRY

Serves: 2 | Prep Time: ~15 min |

Ingredients:

- ½ cup mushrooms (chopped)
- ½ cup cauliflower and broccoli (florets)
- ½ cup asparagus (chopped 1-inch pieces)
- ½ cup green beans
- ¼ cup of red pepper (shredded)
- ¼ cup green pepper (shredded)
- olive oil
- salt and pepper
- 3 tbsp soy sauce

Total number of ingredients: 9

Great salad to consume whenever you're feeling hungry. This salad has a low amount of carbs, but is rich in choline and folates that will increase your histamine and acetylcholine levels.

Directions:

1. In a lightly oiled skillet, add the cauliflower, broccoli, and peppers and let cook for about 5 minutes until softened.
2. Add in the mushrooms, asparagus, and green beans and cook until they are all evenly softened.
3. Add soy sauce and spices and let cook on low heat for 5 more minutes.

WATERMELON AVOCADO SALAD

Serves: 1 | Prep Time: ~10 min |

Ingredients:

- 1 cup watermelon (diced)
- lime juice to taste
- 1 onion (diced)
- ½ avocado (cubed)
- mint, basil, and feta cheese to taste
- 1 tbsp pumpkin seeds
- 2 cups salad greens

Dressing:

- 1 lime's juice
- ¼ cup olive oil
- 1 garlic clove (minced)
- ½ jalapeno (sliced)
- salt and pepper

Total number of ingredients: 13

Another watermelon snack to increase blood flow.
Comes with omega 3 fatty acids.

Directions:

1. Mix all the dressing ingredients and set aside.
2. Mix all salad ingredients, add dressing, and toss.

CHOCOLATE GREEN SMOOTHIE

Serves: 3 | Prep Time: ~10 min |

Ingredients:

- 2 cups spinach
- 2 cups watermelon
- ¼ cup dark chocolate (shredded)
- ½ cup avocado
- 7 ice cubes

Total number of ingredients: 5

Starchy carbs, iron, serotonin and phenyl ethylamine.

Directions:

1. Blend all ingredients until smooth.

ASPARAGUS WITH OYSTER SAUCE

Serves: 4 | Prep Time: ~10 min |

Ingredients:

- 2 tsp vegetable oil
- 1 tbsp ginger
- 2 garlic cloves (minced)
- 1 ½ lb. fresh asparagus (chopped into 2-inch pieces)
- 3 tbsp chicken broth
- 2 tbsp oyster sauce
- ¼ tsp chili flakes
- 1 tsp pumpkin seeds

Total number of ingredients: 8

This recipe helps you boost serotonin and endorphin levels.

Directions:

1. In an oiled skillet, add ginger and garlic until browned, and then add asparagus.
2. Add broth and cook for 5 minutes.
3. Add oyster sauce, pumpkin seeds, and chili flakes and cook for 1 more minute.

STUFFED OYSTERS

Serves: 6 | Prep Time: ~15 min |

Ingredients:

- ◆ 3 tbsp olive oil
- ◆ 1 garlic clove (minced)
- ◆ 10 whole oysters (halved)
- ◆ salt and pepper

For Filling:

- ◆ ½ cup carrot (minced)
- ◆ ½ cup celery root (minced)
- ◆ ¼ cup water
- ◆ ½ cup rice vinegar
- ◆ 2 tbsp chives (minced)

Total number of ingredients: 9

A mix of healthy ingredients. Stays low on carbs.

Directions:

1. Preheat oven to 450 F.
2. In an oiled skillet, place all the "filling" ingredients plus the garlic.
3. Cook on low heat until softened.
4. Place the oysters on a baking tray and carefully lift

each a bit from its shell and add some of the mixture beneath it.

5. Let go of the oyster and place some more filling on the top.

6. Sprinkle with salt and bake for 20 minutes until done.

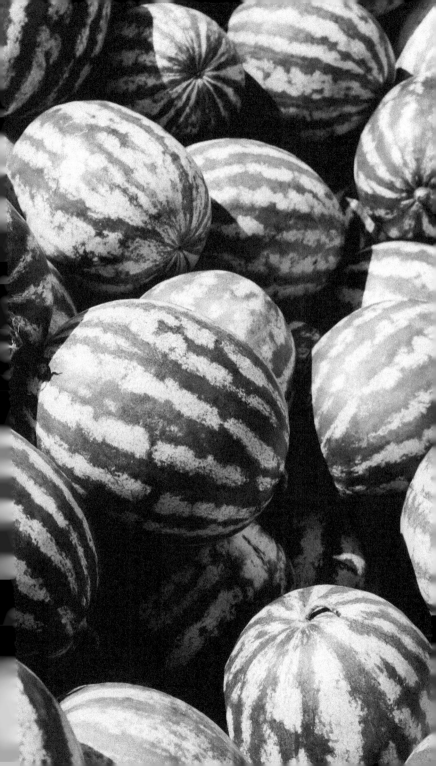

WATERMELON MOJITO (NO ALCOHOL)

Serves: 2 | Prep Time: ~10 min |

Ingredients:

- 10 mint leaves
- 2 tbsps. sugar substitute (Stevia)
- Crushed ice
- ¼ cup fresh lime juice
- 5 oz. seedless watermelon, pureed

Total number of ingredients: 5

Watermelon improves blood flow to both the heart and the rest of your body.

Directions:

1. Mix well in a blender.
2. Serve chilled.

Yogurt Parfait

Serves: 2 | Prep Time: ~10 min |

Ingredients:

- 1 cup of fresh cherries
- vanilla low-fat yogurt
- 2 tbsp flaxseed

Total number of ingredients: 3

Omega-3 fatty acids that come from flaxseeds and saturated fats will improve your testosterone.

Directions:

1. Mix flaxseed with yogurt, then layer yogurt with cherries in a parfait dish.

Spicy Omelette

Serves: 2 | Prep Time: ~10 min |

Ingredients:

- 2 eggs
- 2 tbsp chili peppers, diced or chopped
- 4 tbsp tomatoes, diced
- ½ cup of shredded light emmentaler cheese

Total number of ingredients: 4

Chilies help to increase blood flow and consuming them releases endorphins. Tryptophan from eggs and saturated fats will improve your neurotransmitter production.

Directions:

1. Mix the above ingredients.
2. Place in a frying pan and fry until well cooked.
3. Serve.

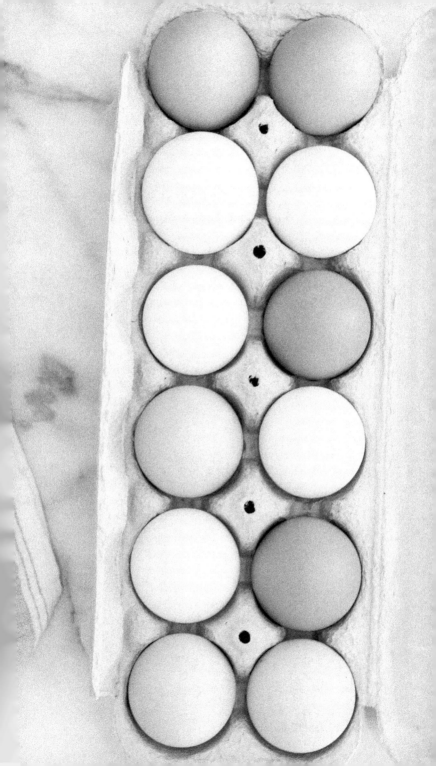

Chocolate Banana Shake / Smoothie

Serves: 2 | Prep Time: ~10 min |

Ingredients:

- Whey protein powder (per directions on package)
- Melted dark chocolate or cocoa powder
- Banana
- Total number of ingredients: 3

Directions:

1. Blend.
2. Serve.

High Protein Oat Cookies

Serves: 48 cookies | Prep Time: ~20 min |

Ingredients:

- ½ cup egg whites
- ¼ cup dark chocolate (shredded)
- 8 scoops vanilla caramel-flavored whey protein powder
- 4 cups oats
- 2 tbsp vanilla extract
- 2 bananas (mashed)
- 4 tsp stevia sweetener
- 2 tsp olive oil
- 1 cup raisins
- ¼ cup of each: walnuts, pecans, and almonds
- 2 tbsp cinnamon
- ½ cup shredded coconut

Total number of ingredients: 14

Whey protein boosts serotonin by moderate amounts. Dark chocolate or cacao powder does the same and contains phenyl ethylamine, the 'love' chemical.

Directions:

1. Preheat oven to 325 F.
2. Mix all ingredients together until smooth.
3. Put on a slightly greased baking sheet and spoon 1tablesoon-sized scoop of batter per cookie.
4. Bake for about 20 minutes.

GREEN PROTEIN SMOOTHIE-

Serves: 1 | Prep Time: ~5 min |

Ingredients:

- 1 cup almond milk
- 1 tbsp ground flax seed
- ¼ cup pecans and walnuts
- 1 scoop whey protein powder
- 1 banana (peeled and frozen)
- 1 cup spinach
- 2 ice cubes

Total number of ingredients: 7

Whey protein boosts serotonin by moderate amounts. On top of that, this recipe contains healthy fats from the nuts.

Directions:

1. Mix all ingredients in a blender and blend until smooth.
2. Serve.

BUCKWHEAT MUFFINS

Serves: 12 | Prep Time: ~15 min |

Ingredients:

- ½ cup buckwheat flour
- 2 tbsp oats
- 1 banana (ripe and mashed)
- ½ cup honey
- 1 tsp cinnamon
- 1 sweet apple of choice (finely diced)
- ½ cup mixed walnuts and pecans (chopped)
- 2 tsp baking powder
- 4 eggs
- ¼ tsp salt

Total number of ingredients: 12

A great serotonin booster.

Directions:

1. Preheat oven to 350 F
2. Line up a 12-cupcake tray with non-stick liners
3. Mix the baking powder, oats, flour, cinnamon, and salt in one bowl, and the banana, honey, and eggs in another.
4. Mix both bowls of ingredients together, then add in the apple and nuts.

5. Spoon into the cupcake liners and allow them to cook for about 30 minutes, or until a toothpick comes out clean.

Sour Cherry Chocolate Smoothie

Serves: 1 | Prep Time: ~5 min |

Ingredients:

- 1 ½ cup almond milk
- ¼ cup sour cherries
- 1 banana (ripe)
- ¼ cup raspberries
- ½ tsp of round flax seeds
- 1 tbsp vanilla whey protein powder
- ¼ cup dark chocolate (shredded)

Total number of ingredients: 7

A perfect drink for your dopamine and serotonin levels. Also provides omega-3s which improve brain functioning.

Directions:

1. Blend all ingredients until smooth.
2. Serve.

Turkey-Egg Casserole with Avocado Slices

Serves: 3 | Prep Time: ~10 min |

Ingredients:

- 3 eggs
- ½ lb. ground turkey
- ¼ cup egg whites
- ½ cup sliced potato
- ¼ cup onion (diced)
- 1 cup spinach
- ½ cup bell pepper (diced)
- 3 tbsp cheddar cheese
- ½ avocado (sliced)

Total number of ingredients: 9

Serotonin booster. The avocado is great for boosting libido. Turkey is a source of tryptophan and glutamic acid that will increase your serotonin and GABA levels.

Directions:

1. Preheat oven to 375 F.
2. In an oiled skillet, cook the turkey and season with pepper and garlic salt.

3. In another bowl, mix the eggs and egg whites and season with salt and pepper.
4. In a deep, lightly oiled baking dish, add a bottom potato layer. Top with another layer of onion, bell pepper, half of the spinach, and turkey. Top with the egg mixture.
5. On top of that, add the cheese followed by the remaining spinach.
6. Cook for about 40 minutes or until the egg layer looks cooked.
7. Cut and serve with sliced avocadoes on the side.

Asparagus Celery Soup

Serves: 6 | Prep Time: ~15 min |

Ingredients:

- 2 tbsp coconut oil
- 2 tbsp celery (chopped)
- 2 garlic cloves (minced)
- salt and pepper
- 4 cups veggie broth
- 1 potato (peeled and cubed)
- 1 lb. asparagus (chopped in 1-inch pieces)
- ¼ cup fresh basil leaves
- ¼ tsp nutmeg
- chives as garnish to taste

Total number of ingredients: 11

A great soup, packed with healthy vitamins, minerals and medium-chain fatty acids to boost neurotransmitter functioning!

Directions:

1. Melt coconut oil in pot and add celery for 3 minutes, then add garlic for about 1 minute.
2. Add in 3 cups of broth and potato and bring to a boil until potatoes are tender.

3. Add asparagus for another 3 minutes the add in the nutmeg, salt, and pepper.
4. Transfer soup to a food processor and blend in the basil, broth, and additional spices.

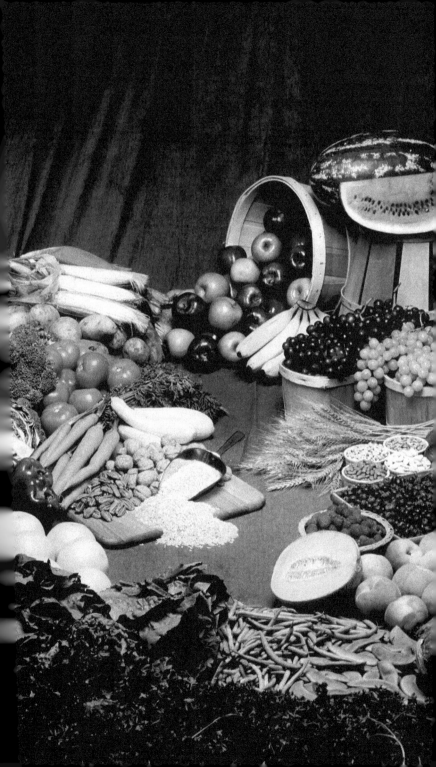

Conclusion

I hope this book was able to help you understand more about adrenal fatigue, what causes it, and most importantly, how to recover from it.

The next step is to begin your journey to health by changing your diet and cutting out the foods that worsen adrenal fatigue and begin eating foods that improve the function of adrenal glands. The only way you can truly make a change is to take massive action. You, and you alone, have to be your own advocate, and I believe you have what it takes to walk the path which so many have, and reclaim the life that you want and deserve. No one is to blame for ending up with adrenal fatigue, but you are 100% responsible for making the changes to create the conditions for your mind and body to nourish your adrenals back to optimum health. I am with you on this journey even if we never meet, I understand how you feel and I promise there is a better way to exist.

CPSIA information can be obtained
at www.ICGtesting.com
Printed in the USA
LVHW040816100320
649438LV00006B/446